F*CK APPROVAL, YOU DON'T NEED IT!

F*CK APPROVAL, YOU DON'T NEED IT!

How to Overcome Approval Addiction and Validate Your Dreams

Elizabeth Moult

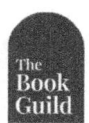

First published in Great Britain in 2025 by
The Book Guild Ltd
Unit E2 Airfield Business Park,
Harrison Road, Market Harborough,
Leicestershire. LE16 7UL
Tel: 0116 2792299
www.bookguild.co.uk
Email: info@bookguild.co.uk

Copyright © 2025 Elizabeth Moult

The right of Elizabeth Moult to be identified as the author of this
work has been asserted by them in accordance with the
Copyright, Design and Patents Act 1988.

All rights reserved. No part of this publication may be
reproduced, transmitted, or stored in a retrieval system, in any form or by any means,
without permission in writing from the publisher, nor be otherwise circulated in
any form of binding or cover other than that in which it is published and without
a similar condition being imposed on the subsequent purchaser.

The manufacturer's authorised representative in the EU
for product safety is Authorised Rep Compliance Ltd,
71 Lower Baggot Street, Dublin D02 P593 Ireland (www.arccompliance.com)

Typeset in 11pt Minion Pro

ISBN 978 1835742 822

British Library Cataloguing in Publication Data.
A catalogue record for this book is available from the British Library.

for my kids
trust your magic &
follow your dreams

CONTENTS

INTRODUCTION		IX
One	**ADMITTING THE TRUTH**	3
Two	**SHIFTING YOUR FOCUS**	25
Three	**RELEASING & LETTING GO**	45
Four	**CONNECTING TO YOUR BODY'S WISDOM**	71
Five	**EMBODIMENT & EXCUSES**	91
Six	**STOP WORRYING ABOUT WHAT OTHER PEOPLE THINK**	114
Seven	**PERMISSION TO GET IT WRONG**	137
Eight	**CLEARING THE RUNWAY TO GET WHAT YOU WANT**	159
Nine	**EMPOWERMENT THROUGH BOUNDARIES & PROTECTION**	182
Ten	**JUST ASK FOR IT**	205
Eleven	**MAGIC IN THE MUNDANE**	227

INTRODUCTION

MOISTURE FILLED THE AIR WITH the scent of the forest as I left the house. The sun hit my skin, an intense reminder of my location, as I made my way to the car. Sunglasses were a must in preparation for when I emerged from the dense subtropical rainforest. Summer days were cool, thanks to the towering gum trees that sheltered the ecosystem below and provided shade around our house. Autumn blue skies sighed with relief at the retreating heat. Winters tested our ability to live frugally, with only six hours of sunlight on our solar panels to provide us with electricity. The wood burner radiated enough heat on those brisk nights that our house was really not built for. Signs of spring would arrive with the intrusion of the local goannas and snakes. Birds and insects orchestrated every ounce of silence, while the fireflies would illuminate the valley and hillside nightly for a precious three weeks. It was pure magic.

We were living the dream. Completely off grid, no phone reception, water from a mountain spring and food from a beautiful communal veggie garden. The beach was a short thirty-minute drive away. You could sit on a headland and watch whales dance in the water, as they migrated along the most easterly point of Australia.

It was the perfect place to raise our children. There was a sense of community, alternative living was normal and I could buy a block of tempeh at my local store. There was space to run wild and run free. Everyone wanted what we had. City folk craved our slow life and the destination, but perhaps not the animals! For a time, we believed that this was what we wanted too.

Arriving at my destination, I had escaped the house in search for something to give my life meaning. I was attending an event to help me to map out my year. I needed to get out of my head, try something new and who knows, perhaps meet some new people. In the beautiful wooden hall, I was surrounded by fifty women; wafts of patchouli and sage perfumed the air; notebooks and yoga mats were at the ready. It was the start of 2021, and the past couple of years had been an epic journey of unravelling my toxic trait of approval addiction. Now I just had to find the final ingredient to close this chapter.

I began journaling in 2017, religiously, most days, to reformat my brain from the bullshit that swirled around it. Some days an easy fifteen-minute session would be enough, while other days I would write for hours, trying to work out why things were the way they were. I was searching for something, putting plans together to change and evolve and 'become better', because I didn't see myself as 'worthy'. Oh, the self-doubt diaries of a disconnected mum who had lost herself to everyone else.

Life should have felt amazing. But it didn't.

INTRODUCTION

I spent most days dragging my feet, pep-talking my sorry ass into making something of myself.

The event began with an hour of meditation and releasing the emotions from the previous year. To say there were tears would be an understatement. I honestly should have packed more tissues, using the bottom of my long skirt to dry my face. I was surprised that apparently I hadn't processed the past few years enough.

Questions were asked. I scribbled down my answers, I felt a surprising sense of calm, and little pressure. But then the big one came. We were asked to write down: what do we want? This boiled down to: what we want for our life, what we want it to look like, no rules, nothing is out of the question and to think beyond what we think we should be writing.

Having someone else ask me these questions allowed me to go into the process, something that I usually controlled. And as I looked around the room I saw so many women who were grateful to be living in this beautiful area. And then it hit me. I wanted out! I wrote – I want to look out of my living room window and see snow-capped peaks and water. I could see this picture in my head, and it made me smile. It made my heart expand. I wanted it.

I left the event straight after this exercise, running to the car listening to the fading squeals of joy as the women I left behind danced in the hall. I was alive. Rushing home, laughing like a crazy lady, I admitted to Roy my husband that I had just left mid workshop to come home to tell him I needed this feeling *to be expanded*, signalling with my arms wide open, more than anything else. Because as much as our cute house was the dream of so many, it had been squashing me from the inside out. It was a cocoon to hide away from the modern world. It had served its purpose but when I looked out of the window all I saw was trees, and I wanted mountains. I know, trees are not a bad thing, but I'm a gal who likes the sky. I like to see clouds moving, stars twinkling. Mountains meant something; we had friends who lived higher than us in the valley and every time I was there, I wanted what they had. It was a deep, unspoken yearning.

The unravelling from the past two years finally revealed something in that journal prompt. A vision that I couldn't let go.

And I didn't care how I was going to make it happen.

I just wanted it so bad.

It was the first time I gave myself permission to admit my dream, no matter how crazy it was.

You see, old Liz would have spent weeks trying to prove to all the people around her why this would be a good idea. Questioning if it was the right thing to do, talking it over endlessly, evaluating, waiting for someone to tell me it was okay to go for it. She would have also spent a lot of that time trying to prove to herself that she could have that thing. WHY? Because she was addicted to approval.

My self-belief had been at an all-time low leading up to that event, moving in and out of depression, dancing with anxiety, and feeling stuck. I felt a constant sickness in my stomach, my head was loud, it stopped me from sleeping, and I was a nervous wreck.

INTRODUCTION

Society feeds us so much garbage about what we should be doing with our lives, and pressures us to tick off lists of achievements. Just so that we can believe that we've done something right. To be seen, to be acknowledged, to gain a sense of achievement.

I had two kids under the age of five; I felt like a shit parent. I was trying to make something out of myself that meant something and I was failing. I felt like a rubbish human. I felt inadequate with most of the people in my life – I felt 'less than' them. Everyone else seemed like they had it all together, big fancy houses, Insta-worthy kids, high-paying jobs and yearly holiday plans. None of that mattered to me. I felt empty. Giving and giving, trying to live up to other people's expectations of me. Somehow I believed I was failing at that too.

But this idea of mountains, and snow and water felt right. *Heart-opening expansion – yesss.*

All I needed was to break the rules. After sharing this with my husband, who had already been looking for jobs, we decided that if this picture was going to be our new reality, he would need to extend his search outside of Australia.

I remember cutting out pictures and sticking them on my wall in my office, laughing it off in disbelief. It didn't seem real to want it. Stupid, in fact. My mind would often chirp in with, *Yeah right, Liz. You're not moving. It's probably a holiday destination only.*

The following week, Roy turned to me while I was cooking in the kitchen to tell me there was a job in Scotland. Butterflies erupted. My stomach dropped. I knew.

F*CK APPROVAL, YOU DON'T NEED IT!

What unfolded over the coming six months was nothing short of remarkable. We moved our family to the other side of the world, to the Scottish Highlands. Remember that vision that I had in my mind when I ran out of that January workshop? Well, that is the view I have from my window; in fact, it's what I am looking at right now. I created that feeling of expansion that I was seeking.

Our family moved during the global pandemic, and amidst state lockdowns, we had to apply to leave our own country. The world was unsettled but we knew a change was needed. The last few years had been wild, but there was a whole new chapter ready to be written.

This experience showed me that anything is possible. That when I trusted myself, I could make magic happen.

I had been living in a place where trying to abide by everyone else's rules made me feel stuck. Don't worry, I also took time to question if I was running away from all my failures. But the truth was, I needed those mountains. I had been fighting my need for approval for over two years, probably longer, practising new ways of living, trying to break free from my head and live from my heart. This move was my ticket to expansion.

Fuck approval, because you don't need it to live the life you desire.

It really has been and continues to be my daily reminder that I don't need anyone's permission to put my happiness first. That I don't need validation. And that I don't need to wait for the life I want to live. Anything is possible – the freedom to be myself, express my feelings, to live life how I want without having to compromise my

INTRODUCTION

values for others. I was no longer willing to wait. I wanted to jump in and drive. I knew I could do it, but I hadn't let myself, because I was full of self-doubt.

I got so curious about my addiction that I studied positive psychology and cognitive behavioural therapy to gain a better understanding of the mind. I knew my body held wisdom but I didn't know how to tune into it. I came to understand that a deep connection to self is an energetic dance between the mind and the body. Once we acknowledge this relationship we begin to truly and freely believe in our own ability to recognise what is right for us. No longer believing anyone who tells us otherwise. That my friend is power.

Stop seeking.

Start believing.

So now I would love for you to see every day as an opportunity. An opportunity to deepen your relationship with yourself, and to investigate, explore, and question everything. Don't worry, I don't expect you to just do it. I am going to walk you through how to do just that over the coming chapters.

Exploring approval addiction, we will look at the role you have been playing in your life, and how you present yourself in different situations. The way you show up for your family might be completely different to how you show up for your friends or in your work. It's important to identify how you adjust yourself for others, and why.

From my story you know that I am now a firm believer in trusting my gut. Who moves their family from Australia to Scotland in a global pandemic? I feel you, it's crazy. And it took a hell of a lot of work to get to a place where I felt confident to back myself. I'm going to shed some light on how the mind–body connection works so you can start to trust your feelings too.

The mind is a powerful machine, and it can either work for you, or against you. I'm going to help you get out of your head once and for all, reduce your anxiety, and teach you how to deal with all the emotions that come out to play. We are saying goodbye to worrying about what other people think.

But look, I'm also a practical-as-fuck country gal, who likes to know how things work. And what every approval-seeker needs to know is how to trust themselves, set boundaries, say no, and ask for help. We go deep with communication and creating healthy relationships. These are all tools I had to practise in order to have the life I have now, one that has me living on the other side of the world, writing daily, hiking and confidently following my desires.

Throughout this book I've included little exercises to support you in living the life you desire without seeking validation. I highly recommend that you take the time to complete each one, in order to transform your life.

Remember, you are not walking this path alone. There are many people who have held themselves back and let others take centre stage. I'm here to remind you that your dreams don't need approval!

Fuck approval!

You don't need it.

Let's do this – it's time to break some rules.

Part One
STOP SEEKING

Chapter One
ADMITTING THE TRUTH

WHEN WE NAME THE PROBLEM... only then can we address it.

Staring up into the rainforest, watching a pair of eagles spiral higher into a thermal, was a welcome distraction as I sat at my desk. It was early 2020, and it had been a week since my life fell to shit. My health was a joke, my stress levels made me defensive about everything, and I had just made the hard decision to cancel a women's conference I was putting together.

I felt like the biggest failure. I was trapped in a constant loop of messy thoughts, analysing every detail of what went wrong.

What could I have done better?

How could I have tried harder?

Why didn't I see it coming?

I've let so many people down. How can I make it up to them?

I had always known this was going to happen but why hadn't I trusted my instincts?

F*CK APPROVAL, YOU DON'T NEED IT!

Sitting in complete disbelief, and nervous anticipation, I was readying myself for a call with Gail, who I was working with to help me write my keynote talk for the event. As I joined the call I was dreading being invited to share with the group about what had been happening. When it came to me, words shot out like toxic lava. It was as if someone had turned on a tap to release the shame that was in me. I felt like I had no control over what was happening.

I spent the first few minutes covering up the epic scale of events that had prevented ticket sales. Bushfires, floods, and now COVID-19. Playing it all down, believing that it was out of my control. Comments were made, geared to seek out confirmation that it had indeed been difficult, and that I was correct that 'it was all doomed' from the beginning. Trying to stay calm, I heard this major confession come out of my mouth. I pretended that I didn't feel like a failure. Who was I kidding?

Mid word vomit, the truth slipped out: 'I left no time for me to talk at my own event.'

A bitter truth even I found uncomfortable admitting. I was working with Gail to prepare my keynote talk and I had forgotten to allocate myself a timeslot. What was the point of even being on this call? To write a talk that I wasn't ever going to make because I had left myself out of the timetable? And now there wasn't even going to be an event, thanks to COVID-19!

I tried to laugh it off and fight back the tears, like it was all nothing. Trying to convince myself I wouldn't let it hurt me.

But it did.

ADMITTING THE TRUTH

Filled with shame and embarrassment, the words 'I did it again' slipped out of my mouth.

Instantly, I stopped talking. White noise filled my brain, I was stunned.

I realised what I had just said out loud. Oh my fucking goodness, I had done this shit before.

My reaction was simply, 'You have got to be fucking kidding me.' I started to kick myself internally. Fuck, fuck, fuck.

How could I have done this to myself?

All I remember was pinching the skin on my leg, trying to stop the deep urge to run and hide.

Embracing the lessons from running the event the previous year, I wanted to speak at this event – to be front and centre, to share my stories – and instead, again, I filled the timetable as quickly as I could with other people, and left myself with nothing.

I didn't prioritise myself. I knew it. All this time, I was putting everyone else ahead of myself. It hurt. Why didn't I listen? Three monumental disasters weren't a big enough sign that I needed to wake up to the truth. Nope, it was the fucking speaker line-up that broke me. As I walked away from the conversation, I had to process how I had even allowed it to happen. It was so darn obvious in retrospect, but at the time I had no clue.

Here I was thinking I was working for the greater good, yet I was driven by an unconscious motivator. I wanted to keep everyone happy. But thanks to my approval addiction, it was totally fucked, and life as I knew it was turned upside down.

F*CK APPROVAL, YOU DON'T NEED IT!

Luckily, Gail caught me after I had dropped mid-sentence into silence. She simply asked, 'You've done this before? How?'

Still mortified, I stared back helplessly in search of something – anything – to get me out of this situation. She suggested that, over the next thirty days, I explore how I was seeking validation from others and to write it down, perhaps as a short story.

My eyes lit up. *Yes.* I went from being a weepy mess on the brink of dying of embarrassment to a butterfly, given permission to spread her wings for the very first time.

All I could think was, *How did she know I wanted to write again?* I missed it. I dreamed of it. It kept popping into my head. But I didn't know what to write. Gail had delivered me a project I could get on board with: writing a journal about my constant need to seek approval from others.

It seemed like a task I could tackle, but I also secretly didn't want to admit to anyone that I, Elizabeth Moult, had consistently let other people walk all over me. I had a persona to live up to, and right now I felt like a total fraud.

Digging right in, I questioned myself endlessly about why I felt like I always needed assurance from others for the things I was doing. The last decade had been filled with days of making sure I was safe from criticism, judgement and failure.

I became consumed by the project that Gail had given me, and I was ready to fill the next thirty days with self-discovery. But thanks to COVID-19, all interaction with the outside world was about to become very limited. Lockdowns now meant that I had to look to my past for the answers. And no one wants to go digging around in there – we push that shit down and away for a reason.

Yet, I persisted.

I wanted to understand why I was always looking for approval – it was like an addiction, an addiction that I was always chasing. Was I an approval addict? Was that it? How could I be? I come across as confident and easy-going. Yet deep down I don't think I ever trusted myself. I was always searching for validation. Validation for who I was, what I was doing, my ideas and even my dreams.

Sound familiar?

Like you, I've secretly second-guessed myself in so many situations. Waiting for a sign that everything is going well, that I've got it right, that I'm doing the right thing. I've even put myself through hell, of my own making, to learn one ridiculous lesson.

You don't need anyone's approval to live your wildest dreams.

TRAITS OF AN APPROVAL SEEKER

Our greatest gift is our awareness, and as approval addicts we are fine-tuned to reading other people. So much so that we usually understand how someone else is feeling before we understand how we are feeling. It's a skill and it's one that we will turn inside out in the next chapter. For now, let's reveal a few truths, shall we? How many of the following approval-seeker traits do you relate to?

F*CK APPROVAL, YOU DON'T NEED IT!

>> *Overly Explaining and Justifying Yourself*

This happens when we doubt ourselves and stuff our truth with long-winded explanations, justifying why things are what they are in the hope that it lives up to the expectation of the receiver. Think talking excessively to get your point across, but in a diplomatic way.

>> *Take on Extra Responsibility*

Nothing says 'I am worthy' more than taking on additional tasks to demonstrate your ability, right? Hard work goes a long way, and being busy is seen as a sign of someone who is living life, who has earned their place.

>> *Not Taking Sick Days*

I always believed I could only take a sick day if I was bedridden, with snot pouring out of my nose, my head pounding, tossing and turning with a fever. I didn't want to let my employers down. I used to push through, proving that I could still do my job under any circumstances – even when it hurt me in the long run.

>> *Fear of Disappointing Others*

You have a strong fear of letting down or disappointing people, which drives many of your actions. As an example, you agree to attend a family gathering you don't want to go to because you don't want to disappoint your parents.

>> *Suppressing Your True Feelings*

You avoid sharing your genuine thoughts and feelings, in order to prevent upsetting or offending others. For instance, you pretend to agree with your partner's political views, even though you have a different perspective, to maintain harmony.

>> *Going Along with the Crowd*

Our desire to fit in drives us to change who we really are; we have all done it. Let's rewind to high school for a moment. Remember those years? Those Reebok Pumps or Doc Martin shoes that you so desperately wanted because all the kids around you had them? Yep, we do this as adults too. It's not just about clothes, but our behaviours too. Perhaps you picked up a new word that you wouldn't normally say? The way you drink your cup of tea? What actions have you adopted simply because it makes you feel like you fit in?

REALITY CHECK

Here is your first dose of tough love. This isn't easy to hear, but if we can get through this bit, we will know where to start to unravel your approval addiction. I spent thirty days digging for stories as to how I was seeking approval and I want you to do the same. Let's talk about journaling for a moment. Writing down your thoughts and emotions makes them real; they become true and, for an approval addict, that can be daunting. Eek! I feel you. I was that person – I didn't want to admit half the things I'm now comfortable about owning.

What if it's wrong? What if I've written it incorrectly? You won't!

Why? Because no one else can tell you how you feel,

or what you are thinking inside your brain. Trust me on this, it will take a week or two for that to sink in and we will talk more about this in another chapter. For now, I want you to start practising being honest with yourself. Own those feelings, own those thoughts, no matter how uncomfortable they are. You are doing this for a damn good reason, because you are done waiting for someone to give you permission to go after your dreams. So…

Here is your journal prompt for the next thirty days. It's tough, but stick with it to find your pattern of addiction.

Thirty-day journal prompt: how/where did I seek out approval today?

What I want you to do is: think about how you said 'Excuse me' ever so politely to the lady in the same aisle as you when you walked by with your trolley, because you would hate for her to think that you were rude or self-important. Yes, that is a form of approval-seeking. If she smiled and nodded, no worries – you would have found your calm again – hello, validation.

Find a moment – a story from your day – where you were trying to please someone's expectations of you by being a good upstanding citizen. I know it's going to take some digging to find these stories, but quite often it's in the little moments where we don't even realise that we are doing it.

With practice you can learn how to catch them.

So, spend about ten to fifteen minutes reflecting over your day. Get that story on a page and begin to understand how your actions were driven by a need for approval.

And if you wish to take it further each day.

Explore who you are seeking approval from.

Why did you need that approval?

What happens once you have got that approval? Think about how it makes you feel or what it might influence.

Just to let you in on a secret, some days I woke up sick to my stomach as another story popped into my head. My tears dripped onto the page as I scribbled down my cringeworthy moments, unforgettable encounters where I was still holding on to rage, blaming others for my own incompetence. My life was fuelled by shame, guilt and fear. How long had I been doing this?

As it turned out, I didn't understand the full scope of my inability to trust myself. I had dressed my own weaknesses as positive attributes – like being kind, super helpful, tough as nails and reliable – all to show others I was good enough.

That month, as I pulled my life apart to uncover my truth, I began to recognise my behaviours and habits. Discovering the 'how' helped me to admit my most familiar patterns and allowed me to see that I had needs too. The threads were all interlinked. Some of the signs were obvious while others took a little digging. To be honest, I didn't want to acknowledge my part in any of them.

THE APPROVAL TRAP

Approval addiction is where we seek out validation to justify our self-worth.

As humans, we love helping others because it makes us feel good. We are a collective of social creatures who thrive in communities. We go about our daily lives strengthening our bonds through acts of kindness and generosity. We love nurturing others because seeing them thrive gives us the warm and fuzzies.

We all want to feel useful because it gives us a sense of purpose.

However, when our acts of kindness come from a place of wanting acceptance, seeking approval, needing validation, needing to feel loved, or to avoid fear, it's not kindness anymore. It's people-pleasing, in which we're doing these 'kind' things to alter or even manipulate a situation.

Kindness is giving from a full cup, where we have the ability to give without expectations, judgement or assumptions.

When we feel any resentment or frustration after performing an act of kindness, it most likely means that we are in fact trying to please the other person.

Now, it's not to say we should stop being kind, because that's not what this is about. It's about knowing when we go above and beyond at the cost of our own happiness.

People-pleasing is when we sacrifice ourselves to avoid feelings of discomfort while not wanting to let others down. It's working to live up to *their* expectations, avoid hurting *their* feelings or proving our worth to *them*, all without thought to what it's doing to us. As approval addicts, our actions are geared towards others' reactions. We worry about how we will be seen, or interpreted, and if we will be accepted. We give and give, waiting for something in return. But at the end of the day, the only person who is going to make you happy is you!

It's time to end the approval trap and trust yourself. So, let me ask you this: do you like helping others?

Is it because you like the feeling you get when you do it?

Do you do it because you genuinely want to see the other person thrive?

Do you do it because you feel like you are contributing to something greater?

Or do you do it out of fear, shame or guilt?

The fact that you want to see others happy is completely normal. Please don't stop being kind. More people should be kind and treat others like they themselves would like to be treated. But there is a point where our generosity becomes compromised, and it's important for us to know where the need to help comes from. Remember, it's healthy to do acts of kindness but not at the cost of your happiness.

We should never feel resentment about helping others. And if we do, that is our cue to open up an investigation and take a good hard look at our own behaviours.

DIGGING UP THE PAST

My past revealed way more than I had realised or been willing to admit. It wasn't pleasant. That's why people call it 'the work'. When I was journaling each day, I was dredging through stories that I thought were normal, nit-picking and justifying my actions. So I decided to seek out support from a professional and expanded my studies because I needed to more deeply understand the WHY...

What I came to learn and understand is that, as children, the people around us help paint the picture of the roles we play in life. They show us how to treat others, how to treat ourselves, how to care for our homes, and what it means to work, live and play.

F*CK APPROVAL, YOU DON'T NEED IT!

I had a friend who was mind-blowingly ambitious. She spoke on large international stages with a grand vision. I loved her for it; she had that 'zest for life'. I attended a workshop she was leading and it hit me that I was playing down my own capabilities out of fear of what she would think. I honestly thought I stood by her side as an equal. But what I discovered was that I saw her as an authority figure. She was here to teach me, and show me the way, instead of all this 'self-enquiry, find the answers for yourself' business. You could say I was pretty pissed at my discovery.

Taking this information to my therapist, we explored why I kept reverting back to the role of a small child, looking up to those around me as far mightier. Everyone around me – teachers, parents, government, bosses, police officers, mentors, doctors – they were all authority figures in my life. Their role was to keep me safe and show me how I was supposed to live. So I stood to attention and did what they said.

Fearful of doing something wrong, I had a real aversion to them at the same time. Yet I kept them happy by getting great grades, doing overtime at work, not getting into trouble, staying out of the way, and not speaking up. The list goes on. And I bet I am not the only one who has fallen into this pattern. Think about it. When you were a small child, your parents were your caretakers. They were the ones that provided your security in life – home, food, love, guidance, and protection. Relying on them to nurture your needs, they were your 'almighty big people'. During these years you created responses to their actions/needs in order to see the smile on their face, and to be rewarded with a hug, or get a treat. This was the beginning of your approval addiction.

As we grow up, there are those who spread their wings with a sense of freedom, and those who continue to seek validation that what we are doing is right.

When I was in my mid-twenties, I had a job as a chef at a luxury retreat venue. I was in charge of the kitchen, until one day a new staff member became the person to report to. She came with enthusiasm and an endless list of suggestions. She nurtured me, helped with tasks, and one day, all of a sudden, I felt like I was no longer in charge. She had come in and stamped her authority in my space, and I had immediately abided by what she said, instead of trusting myself. Now, I was constantly second-guessing everything.

The relationship became strained, and it wasn't until I had an Emotional Freedom Technique (tapping) session with a colleague that we worked out that I saw her as someone greater than me. I had responded to her by becoming small in the scenario; I was not her equal, and I felt helpless, stuck, and not heard. We were both grown women, but I reverted back to being a child in the relationship. In my world, that meant I abided by the rules, tried not to upset people, and avoided conflict.

These scenarios are all too common for approval addicts, so why does this happen?

BEING SMALL (PLAYING THE ROLE OF A CHILD)

When we feel small, we revert back to the role of a child. This is where we consider ourselves as vulnerable, with a desire to be nurtured and feel the need to guard ourselves.

In the diagram below is how we perceive ourselves in the childlike state when we don't see others as equal to us. We deem the other person – parents, partners, colleagues, bosses, teachers, friends or any authority figure – as far superior.

This response, taking on the role of a child as an adult, can be a self-defence mechanism to keep us safe from being hurt. It's a learned behaviour from our early childhood, where we feared getting it wrong, or letting people down. We were worried we wouldn't get the love we craved. We didn't get the protection we needed or the guidance to stand on our own feet. Instead, we were taught to follow the rules, to be upstanding citizens who don't get in trouble.

Before you get all fired up about finding someone to blame, take a breath.

This is a learned behaviour – you did this. It sucks to hear it, but honesty is key here.

It's always been your responsibility to grow and learn – you might have just learned some unhelpful stuff along the way.

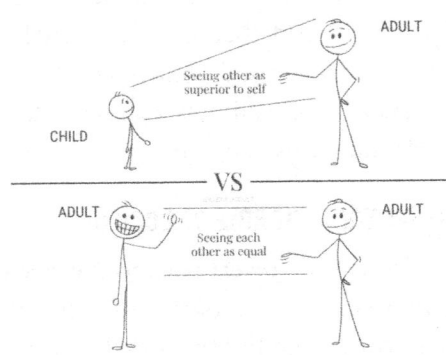

SEEING OURSELVES AS EQUAL (ROLE OF AN ADULT)

In order to see ourselves as an equal, we need to strip away all our beliefs about what makes the other person superior. It's hard to admit that we have taken on the role of 'child' in this scenario, but we all do it from time to time.

There comes a point during childhood, adolescence, and maturity when we learn to communicate with people in our own way. If we experience a disruption in our development, it stalls the process. When we are nurtured to maturity to think, express, and communicate our needs, we become more self-assured, which is not a bad thing.

Yes, you may have judgements about those who know how to ask for what they want. In actual fact, these people hold the magic of self-trust, even though we might want to sneak in and label them as 'lucky', because nothing is holding them back.

Approaching others with the knowledge that the other person is the same as us – a human being with emotions, feelings, reactions, and a repertoire of responses that they too created while growing up, as well as problems that aren't always visible on the surface – should not equate to changing who we are. It's about standing side by side, and not adjusting our own identity.

REWRITING THE RULES

Approval addiction destroys our true self and prevents us from shining. It keeps us waiting constantly for validation that may never come. Our self-worth is always scanning for breadcrumbs. We are in fact living by the rules of others, at the mercy of a validation handout, to fill that little gap that needs a hit, in order to reassure us that we are in the correct place. So, it's time to address a few home truths.

When I think of 'rules', I get a bit cringy. No one likes being told what to do. I hear you!

I'm a gal who went to art school and apparently you need to learn the rules, in order to break them, in order to create good art. Well, I want you to take on this philosophy for a moment. As kids we learned how to be good humans thanks to our parents either role-modelling, teaching or showing us how.

In our house my mum did most of the cooking, my grandmas were renowned for their cakes and bread, and I took it as my responsibility to learn this skill too. Being a helper meant that I got to learn the terminology of the kitchen. Pass me the salt, get the milk, find the flour, turn on the oven and have you seen the baking tray?

All normal stuff. I was curious; I wanted to learn and so I did. I went to the people who demonstrated skills, who could show me the way. When I was eighteen, I lived in a shared house, where I had two very keen helpers when it came to making dinner. They had no cooking skills whatsoever. One day while making the house 'fave' – bangers and mash – I was searching frantically in the utensils drawer as they stood in the doorway filling me in with the latest gossip. I yelled for help, 'Where are the pinchy things?' Laughter erupted immediately. I was getting flustered at the thought of burning dinner while the discussion of what the hell 'pinchy things' were took the spotlight.

The thing with breaking the rules is – it doesn't have to

be huge. All my life I believed that a pair of kitchen tongs were called 'pinchy things'. Who was I to question what was normal, because that was all I knew. Slightly embarrassing to admit that an eighteen-year-old believed that they lived alongside the flippy-over-doover – go figure.

At this young age, I started to question my truth. What was real and what wasn't.

Many start this journey around twelve years old; me, eighteen. The idea is that we challenge the normal, we challenge what we have been taught and come to our own decisions about life. Many adults wonder why teenagers are so rebellious. Well, let me tell you, they are trying to work out their truth and how they fit into society, stretching, flexing and testing things out. It's challenging to establish a sense of place. This rite of passage is a vital opportunity to question life and themselves. Remember that desire to feel like we belong? This is a crucial time to test those boundaries, those rules and to get caught doing something we know we shouldn't be doing.

Well, what if we apply that to today?

Did the fear just creep in a little at the thought of breaking the rules?

Yes, breaking the rules comes with its own consequences, but with a little hindsight they can be packaged up as life lessons. Not all rule breaking leads to chaos, jail sentences or worse, being sent to your room!

I want to channel a little Taylor Swift for a moment – I did something bad, but why does it feel so good?

Eek, the first time you stand up for yourself is a moment you will never forget.

F*CK APPROVAL, YOU DON'T NEED IT!

In late 2005 I was desperately working three jobs to make some cash. I had only been back in Australia for two months and was still paying off the last of my expenses from living abroad. The first job I secured was with my old job. My boss loved me, and I knew she would give me a job, because this approval seeker worked hard, and demonstrated that she was awesome at what she did. It took years of overtime, Christmas shifts and covering people calling in sick to earn her trust and get to this place. But I did it.

Juggling jobs is never easy, but I had a goal in mind – it was my first business idea. Travelling had given me so many life lessons, and made me question everything about myself, and the world we live in. It had been completely eye-opening, so I knew I didn't want to settle for just anything.

When a friend suggested I apply to work at her bar – where they paid overtime after 8pm, Saturday was time and a half and Sunday was double – it was an easy yes. More money, working less time. It was a no-brainer.

Yet guilt came up. Thinking about how to tell my boss, who had given me a job as soon as I got home, that I was leaving made me feel sick. It was like I owed her something. I was her go-to for extra shifts, extra hours when someone was off sick. I was never sacked. I was re-hired as soon as I asked. See, now I'm proving to you how awesome I am, ha-ha-ha.

Take a moment here. There are times when it's great to gloat about our successes, but in this little life lesson, I had to break up with the rule 'being loyal is more important than my happiness'.

I did it. I gave notice after only working six weeks, for something better, something that meant I could do more with my life.

Was I breaking the rules? Yes! Because…

I believed that one should be loyal to people.

I believed that I should work hard for them to earn their trust.

I believed that I had to work hard to earn money.

I believed that if I let someone down, it was burning a bridge and that relationship would be over.

What happened after I created more space and freedom was that I set up art classes, taught life drawing, and ran exhibitions. I've always loved art, and still paint today. That business was a huge success; I was able to see it when my next evolution took place.

But, if I hadn't created that space by taking the job with fewer hours for more money, if I hadn't questioned what I believed and if I'd remained living up to the expectations of what I thought others thought of me, life would have turned out very differently.

So here is what we are going to do next. Think of this as clearing space to make room for new possibilities, by letting go of the rules you are living up to that no longer serve you.

Burn the Rule Book: A Clearing Ritual

As you start to collect your stories of approval seeking, it's important to remember that they are not what are going to define you as you move forward. You have the opportunity to rewrite the rules and to let go of the past. This ritual

F*CK APPROVAL, YOU DON'T NEED IT!

is about opening yourself up to 'anything is possible'. It's about removing the limitations you have settled on in the past, and have lived by, that no longer put your happiness front and centre. It's time to reclaim some space for the new to come in, and break free from the approval trap of old rules.

Let your inner teenager out here for this ritual; channel some rebellious vibes.

Step 1: Prepare Your Sacred Space

Find a quiet place where you feel safe and grounded. This could be in your home, a garden, or anywhere that feels personal to you. Bring a piece of paper, a pen, matches, or lighter, and a fireproof container or bowl to safely burn your paper.

Set the intention that this space is dedicated to your growth and release. You may want to light a candle, play calming music, or have any items around that make you feel grounded, such as crystals or meaningful objects.

Step 2: Reflect on the Rules You've Lived By

Take a deep breath and centre yourself. Reflect on the stories you have been writing – what beliefs, habits, and unspoken rules dictated your approval-seeking behaviour/habits.

Think about the moments where you:
- *Made yourself small in the presence of others.*
- *Changed who you were, to fit in.*
- *Said 'yes' when you meant 'no'.*
- *Hid your true self, for fear of rejection.*

ADMITTING THE TRUTH

Allow these rules to surface. Some might be clear and obvious, while others may be subtle or ingrained. Write them down as they come to you.

Examples of Limiting Rules:

- *'I must always keep others happy, or they won't love me.'*
- *'I can't speak my mind because I'll hurt people.'*
- *'If I'm not perfect, I'll be judged.'*
- *'My worth depends on what others think of me.'*

Be honest. This is your space to express the rules that no longer serve you.

Step 3: Write

Once you've written your rules down, read them aloud. Notice how they make you feel. Is there tension? Relief in acknowledging them? Do they still feel true to you?

Is there more you need to say about these rules? Start with one, and write the story of when and where this was true in your life. Who was there, what happened, how did you feel, why did you take this rule on as your own? Thoughts and emotions matter here the most. Get it out. Even if you need to write the word 'Fuck' fifty-three times to get your point across, to explain how upset and angry you are about it – do it! This is about liberating that approval seeker who doesn't like to get it wrong. I was taught not to swear but golly when I do, it is so intended. Feel through it. Tell that rule where you want to shove it and how you never want to see it again.

Step 4: Release

Next, it's time to release them. Hold the piece of paper and say the following:

'I acknowledge these rules for what they are – limitations from my past. They have served me in some way, but I no longer need them. I am ready to let them go and live by my truth.'

With intention, carefully light the paper and place it in the fireproof container. As the paper burns, visualise these rules dissolving. Imagine the weight lifting off your shoulders as they transform into ash and smoke, released into the universe.

Expect a tear, especially if you have collected a few pages to burn at once. This is big! You are ready to reclaim your essence, and your soul's truth.

Step 5: Reflect and Reclaim

Once the paper has burned completely, take a few deep breaths and sit with the energy of release. You've made a conscious decision to let go of rules that no longer serve you.

Blow out any candles, take one last deep breath, and feel the new space you've created within.

This is not a one-time process. You may discover new rules as you continue on your journey, and that's perfectly okay. The key is to recognise when these rules begin to limit you, so that you can let them go, and reaffirm your truth.

Every time you clear space, you make room for more of your authentic self to shine. To do that, we need to shift our focus away from pleasing others, and towards pleasing ourselves. Turning our awareness inside out. Your addiction won't know what's happening.

Chapter Two
SHIFTING YOUR FOCUS

I USED TO BE A rebel. I was the girl at the party who would waltz into a room and have everyone in awe, their attention and curiosity caught by my presence. I felt it; they felt it; it was magnetic. I loved it – I had become the girl I always wanted to be.

The music was loud, and pumping through our makeshift stereo, which, despite the amount of gaffer tape and cable ties holding it together, surprisingly worked. People filled every corner, from the lounge to the hallway to the downstairs toilet. With smoke-filled air, and enough booze for at least another one hundred people, this was the norm in our shared house; it was a Friday in 2009, and it deserved to be celebrated. With too many drinks under my belt, I was having a great time, but knew I needed to eat something.

My failsafe way to keep the partygoers fed was to drunkenly make a batch of popcorn. It helped me to have something in my belly before passing out after a night of wild

F*CK APPROVAL, YOU DON'T NEED IT!

drunken stories, board games (which of course had been turned into drinking games) and dancing. All the while, chain-smoking like a trooper. I pulled out the largest pot that had a lid that actually fitted, poured in some oil, and placed it on the stove. While I waited for it to heat up, I rolled a ciggy and smoked at least half of it while I leaned against the bench. As the oil began to smoke, I tipped in the corn kernels, and put the lid on. Waiting for the first popping sound, my moment of peace was interrupted by Stacey, a friend of a friend.

We started off with the usual light conversation stuff, but then she said, 'Why do you act the way that you do?'

Completely dumbfounded by this question, I played along. 'Mmmm-hmm right, okay.' The corn started to pop, and I turned away from her to shake the pot, hoping she would leave or change the subject.

But as I worked my magic over the stove, Stacey kept on with the questions, leaning over my shoulder in her perfectly curated outfit that would have suited Rachel from *Friends*. We weren't particularly close – in fact we hadn't had very many conversations of substance. Yet here she was explaining to me that nobody liked how I was always trying to prove myself. 'It's unnecessary,' she told me. 'Especially when you're trying to show off with your stories. It's like you want to prove you're better than the rest of us.'

The popcorn fell silent and I pulled it from the stove, shaking in disbelief. 'What do you mean?' I asked, my voice ever so trembly.

Oh, Stacey went on and on, while I stood there and took it all. I dominated conversations, and that was not cool. Sometimes I was a bit of a dickhead.

My insides started to burn up. 'I don't tell stories to be better,' I said, trying to justify myself.

But she just doubled down on her opinion, telling me again, 'You don't need to prove yourself all the time. Nobody likes it! It's super annoying and totally not necessary.'

Did she think she was helping me? Did she think I would appreciate the feedback, and thank her for her brutal honesty? Cornered and shaken, I looked for an escape route as tears began to well in my eyes. I tried to hold it all in. The popcorn was the excuse I needed to get the hell out of there, so I ferried it around the house as quickly as I could, just so I could lock myself in my room to process what the fuck had just happened. I felt so helpless. My mind was spiralling out of control. What had I done that was so wrong? How could it be that people – who I thought were my friends – *didn't* like me at all?

It hurt. It hurt so deeply. This shared house was the first place in my life where I had felt able to be completely 'me'. I felt like I belonged, and people accepted me. But now, thanks to Stacey's inside information, I discovered that they only tolerated me, and found me rather annoying. It triggered the shit out of me. I was suddenly an outsider.

I fell across my milk-crate double bed as the party kept going outside. I released a big hot mess of tears that streamed down my face, gasping for air. I was so, so angry and upset. I wondered if I really was a shit person.

Alone, and with my safety net pulled out from underneath me, I felt like I had no one to talk to. Surrendering into my blubbering, I didn't sleep a wink.

F*CK APPROVAL, YOU DON'T NEED IT!

I went over the scenario again and again, making myself even more miserable. I was my own worst enemy.

Did I hate Stacey for what she said? No, of course not.

Did I hate everyone for not saying something? No, of course not.

Did I hate myself? Hands down, a big fat yes.

How could I have let this happen? The birds chirping outside my window reminded me that it was time to get the fuck up. It was a new day. All I could think was, *Okay, who did I need to become to avoid this ever happening again?*

My solution was that *I* needed to change.

I could no longer be myself. This is what my logical mind came up with, anyway.

There could be no more obnoxious, drunk Liz. I had to control my behaviour because I couldn't trust that I wouldn't be a dickhead. I got out of bed and declared that I wasn't drinking ever again – health kick, you know? I couldn't share the real reason why, let alone what had been said the night before. It was embarrassing. I walked around the house with my head down because knowing that my people thought I wasn't good enough forced me to push every ounce of myself away, including my feelings.

I moved with absolute care. I was acutely conscious of everything around me, from people to how loud the music really got, to the slurring conversations that didn't go anywhere. My eyes were wide open for the first time when someone started telling a story that went round and round in circles and ended up back at the beginning, just to repeat itself all over again. When someone spits unknowingly as they make their point, spraying all those people listening around them, I wondered, *Was I one of those people?*

All of a sudden, I was agonisingly aware. I, too, was a bad drunk, with my expressive storytelling arms, my dance moves, my opinions and my general need for people to acknowledge me. It was confirmed: Drunk = Bad.

I spent a lot of time hiding the truth. Stacey's words had hit me hard like a brick to the face. I crafted a new set of rules to live by in order to keep the peace. I loved where I lived, I loved the people, but I was so hurt at the thought of them not liking me. I didn't know what else to do except to pretend that I didn't know. To keep going, and adjust who I was, so that I wasn't seen as annoying, and someone that they wouldn't like.

Several months later, the first drink after my detox hit me hard. The impact of the alcohol running through my veins lit me up, and my face started to burn. I was high on sugar, and I was nervous. Back then I didn't know what anxiety was, or even how it played out. Right after that one drink, I drank three cups of water to make up for the poison running through me, hoping to dilute the effects. Maybe it wouldn't be noticeable.

After all, I wanted to blend into the crowd. I didn't want to be seen like I had been before. This was Liz 2.0 and she was different. She wasn't the life of the party; she was a cool cat who clung to the walls.

It was hard at first to bite my tongue. I felt like I was a kid again, having to watch what I said and did. The thought of not being liked outweighed the heaviness I felt in my heart.

F*CK APPROVAL, YOU DON'T NEED IT!

I no longer trusted myself.

Every week threw another challenge at me, and soon I started to feel like I didn't belong anymore. I became the joke at parties, and my so-called friends teased me and pulled faces when I did talk. I tried to not take it on, but it felt like high school all over again.

I became super sensitive and hyper-vigilant. I was consistently anticipating situations, trying to figure out what people might say or do so that I could try to please them. I would even apologise for being me. I walked on eggshells, with friends, family, and workmates. I stopped going to parties and social events because it was so uncomfortable. I couldn't relax the ticking time bomb of nerves I held inside.

Broken, I kept myself guarded and hid myself away from the world. For those who were still in my life, I went above and beyond, trying to seek their approval by not putting them out by simply being me.

It was hard work!

If only I could go back to that moment and remind myself that it doesn't matter what people think, and that one person's thoughts about me are not something that I need to take on. I would tell my past self that their reaction to me was a reflection of their own beliefs and insecurities.

The irony in my story is somewhat hilarious. I became an approval junkie because someone told me I was working too hard to prove myself. It triggered me so much that I shut down and became more concerned about what others thought of me than how I thought of myself.

Hitting the fast-forward button, I can clearly see how I

went from living a carefree life to instantly entertaining a torturous dialogue, fuelled by self-doubt.

In this chapter we are going to explore the intricacy of the mind and the inner critic, exploring how it rolls and why it pipes up with nasty-ass comments. We are going to address why it's so easy to look out from ourselves as approval addicts, and not look within. By the end of this chapter, I want you to be able to recognise your internal BS and how the outside world plays a role in keeping you away from your wildest dreams.

THE INNER BITCH & HER QUEST

I would have given myself a Golden Globe for the monologue that I produced at times. I seriously knew how to tear someone down. The only problem was that I was doing it to myself. It's time for you to meet your Inner Critic – the inner bitch who lives in your head, and who is on a quest to keep you there too.

The mind is powerful, and it's the home of the Inner Critic. The Inner Critic shares the space with a lot of other important functions, like keeping you moving and physically balanced, problem solving, processing new and existing information, and most importantly translating feelings and sensations into words.

It's pretty wild when you realise just how much power the mind has over us. Humans have somewhere between fifty to seventy thousand thoughts a day; that is an information superhighway running at lightning speed. To me, that just sounds exhausting. No wonder there are so many of us walking around in a mind funk on a daily basis, feeling stuck, frustrated and at a loss about how to move forward.

It's so bloody noisy.

However, not all thoughts are created equal. Some are loud and demand attention while others slip past in an instant.

And this is where it gets interesting.

We are constantly accumulating information, day in, day out, processing what is important and what is not. Our mind filters everything around us. It's a basic system with some information getting stored while other observations pass us by.

Our brains use this gathered information to respond from an informed place of acquired knowledge.

VALIDATION IN ACTION & WHY THE OUTSIDE WORLD IS DANGEROUS AF!

When we go out into the world each day to tackle life, we are giving our body information to process. As you may now understand, the brain is epic. As approval addicts, our brains are wired to focus on others first. We want to assure them. And we want to feel some form of validation, that what we are doing is right. So, let's break this down a bit further.

When I first started socialising again after the kitchen incident, I had my eyes open wide. I saw things I had never seen before. I was so self-conscious. The smallest of gestures could signal if I was doing something right or wrong.

If I stood next to a particular person and started talking to them, I would assess the vibe. I would first check if that person was okay with me saying hello. Did they greet me with kindness, and take an interest in what I had to say? Computing that information, I would then either continue with a conversation, or move away and try something else.

The outside world fed my Inner Critic confirmation regularly. With statements like – *Yep, you're right, they don't like you, there is no point.*

My Inner Critic was working against me. She tore me down. She was setting me up!

The outside world feeds us rules to live by all the time. Social standards about how to be good. What we should aim for in life. The things we need to acquire to be successful. The material world is driven by a marketing machine that prays on approval addicts, because we want validation that we made it, got it right. That new house, new car, new watch, it all seems pretty epic. But here is the thing – now that you've got the thing you worked so damn hard for, do you still feel empty? Did anyone acknowledge or approve of you reaching that milestone?

Gah, I hate to confess it. I remember buying a dress for one hundred dollars – it was a huge investment from me, completely out of my budget. But I wanted to look the part when I went to a wedding and it brought me a small moment of happiness. But after the wedding the dress sat in my cupboard, never to be worn again. I was constantly being pressured by the people around me that I had to make an effort in the wardrobe department – it was going to be fancy. People confirmed my lack of style, and I wanted to prove them wrong. I was desperate to live up to their expectations. The dress was totally not me. I looked the part, but I still felt separate from everyone else.

This is why it's important to understand that what the outside world feeds you needs further investigation. It's not just because someone told you so. Oh, I just had a knee-jerk reaction to that. Did anyone else have a moment from childhood where a parent told you something and you asked *why* and their response was, 'Because I told you so'?

This is the start of rule-making and confirming that you are not in charge of your life. THEY ARE.

If you remember from the previous chapter how authority figures play a significant role in our life, it's no wonder the outside world is dangerous – it's us versus them. And there are a lot of 'them' out there.

THE MIND WANTS US TO STAY SAFE

Humans crave security. After thousands of years, we still seek safety even though we live in a world with far fewer threats than our ancestors. We all want to have a roof over our heads, food in our bellies, clothing on our backs, money in our accounts and love in our hearts. These are our basic essentials for a comfortable life.

This is the Inner Critic's quest. She's just trying to keep you safe!

Or is she…?

Our minds create patterns to prevent us from steering into unfamiliar territory. I spent most of my childhood as the black sheep. I was always the different one, the weird one, the difficult one, the drama queen, the one who was 'too much'. That moment in the kitchen triggered me back to square one. The feeling of belonging I had was taken away from me in a second.

I put on a brave face to keep going each day. Instead of challenging what Stacey said, I decided that it was safer if I retreated. Why? Because that was what I knew. My Inner Critic knew all the right things to keep me away from being hurt further, from being judged more harshly, and even worse, being ignored and cast out.

Doing something new or different is uncomfortable. It triggers the alarm bells in our brain because it doesn't have the required information to process how things will turn out. It's unfamiliar. And so, the mind sees it as potentially not safe.

We used to have a flock of fifty chickens and they do this too! We had a chicken that got a little sick, and within a day she dropped to the bottom of the pecking order. I had a soft spot for her, so I gave her extra food and attention. I felt her weakness, but the thing is with chickens and a lot of animals, even when they are sick, they pretend they are okay in order to survive. If they show any signs of weakness, they are outed from the rest of the group. Sometimes it's pretty much a death sentence. It's a cruel world, and it can be the same for us humans. History is a dark place. But this instinct to survive is in us too. We want to blend in and not be 'outed' or seen as weak or inferior.

Stretching myself would have been an act of bravery. I would have said – Fuck Approval, You Don't Need It – and especially not from Stacey – who does she think she is? My storytelling is amazing and it makes me who I am! Don't let her take that away from me.

I love me a pep talk.

Avoiding discomfort is what our mind helps us to do. Yet, in doing this, we miss opportunities to expand and enrich our lives. Some challenges come with greater risk, while with others, we kick ourselves for not doing them earlier.

So, we need to have a moment here with the Inner Critic.

The Inner Critic warns you off from exploring uncharted territory. It also turns into a bit of a bitch and tears you down when you have done something wrong, because you created rules for yourself. We are going to explore this in another chapter.

This loud dialogue can be all-consuming. I've been there, I spent a good forty-eight hours working out how to deal with that kitchen incident and I got so stuck in my head. I couldn't move, I just felt physically stuck, I cried my heart out on the bed. I let my Inner Critic win. She knew that my relationship with self-doubt and my fear of not belonging would hurt me. She knew it was me that had to change (so she had come to believe – ah, how naive I was) because I was the problem.

Me! I was the problem.

The dreaded approval-addict curse! Not living up to other people's expectations. I lived in my head for a decade trying to adjust to others to get their approval. My brain lived for this information; it's how I created some of the rules I live by.

I'm not sure what would have happened if I had decided to do something different. I'm not going to dwell on it, because it's in the past. I can't go back and magically fix it. Unless you know someone who's got time travel skills that could help me out? Yet, when we make these decisions, we always have an opportunity to fine-tune the outcome. I stayed in it for years, created a whole new rule book focused on others – far away from what I really wanted.

I don't want you to make my mistake and make it your new normal.

I became an approval addict because I didn't trust that I was enough as I was. Yep, a whole lot of self-doubt going on.

Living in my head was exhausting, it wears you down and it stops you from exploring new possibilities. It's where the Inner Critic is playing dirty. Bitch! And the thing we really need to do is fact-check those thoughts. To check if they are valid.

So it's time to run our Inner Critic's opinions through the ringer.

And sometimes it helps to give it a name – many of my clients have adopted the inner bitch or you could try: the bad bitch, bitchass, bitch face, brain-bitch or negative Nancy.

Fact Checking

Fact checking is our opportunity to qualify our thoughts. It puts life into perspective in the present moment. It stops us drowning our thoughts. The best time to use it is when your Inner Critic is tearing you down. Cause she ain't right all the time!

F*CK APPROVAL, YOU DON'T NEED IT!

Address your most repetitive thought...

What does my inner-critic say to keep me from breaking the rules and staying small? Write down your thought.

_____
_____
_____
_____
_____
_____

Is this thought I'm having true?

_____
_____
_____

Is it useful for me to think about it?

_____
_____
_____

Does this thought add value to my life?

_____
_____
_____

Who's voice is this?
(Is it mine or someone else's?)

_____
_____
_____

Where did I learn this from? (Dig deep into the story behind where you picked it up.)

_____
_____
_____
_____

SHIFTING YOUR FOCUS

Do you still believe it now? Is it still true? If so, why?

This exercise is great to address those pesky one liners that fly around in our head, from excuses to why we are not enough. It challenges the way you think instead of accepting your life as it currently is.

Let's Get Curious

Luckily our minds are super curious. They love to learn. We just need to stay open to freely absorb new information. Then it's up to us to process the information we have acquired, so we can shift the output to our new way of being.

So I want to ask you…

What would you do if you were brave?

Use that sentence as a journal prompt. Challenge your Inner Critic. If you were in my situation, what would you have done if you were brave? I decided to run and hide, to stay safe. I wasn't brave at all, but if I had asked that question, I think my life would have changed significantly, and I wouldn't have this story to tell and that is why we can't dwell on the past. I've got my scars and battle wounds and I've learned loads from them. I am richer for it.

F*CK APPROVAL, YOU DON'T NEED IT!

Living in our mind sucks. The weight is heavy, especially when it's stuck in a negative loop. Rules to follow and live by. Expectations to live up to. They were formulated from past life events, patterns and behaviours that were fine-tuned to keep us from being hurt. Yay for learning, but it's important to challenge those rules from time to time.

I will never forget the day when my flatmate Mark walked out of a yoga class after ten minutes because it wasn't his jam. I was gobsmacked. Not only did I feel bad for dragging him there in the first place, but I felt bad because he struggled with the fast-moving sequences. Yet he was totally chill about it. He knew it wasn't for him, so he got up and walked the fuck out of there as if it was nothing. No approval required. He changed his situation.

He was brave.

Approval seeking lives in the mind. It's those expectations, judgements and behaviour patterns that we have formulated to keep us safe, and to keep our life in balance. Yet when we get our mind on board with what our body's craving, we can take deliberate bold steps forward. We can rewrite our future instead of living in the same loop that keeps playing over and over again. My friend Mark knew his body was not going to handle that hectic yoga class, so why stay? Why persevere just to be polite? Fuck polite.

He didn't give a shit about what other people thought.

He left because he knew his body, and its capabilities.

He wasn't living up to anyone's expectations but his own.

That's the kind of attitude I want: to know my body but also to take action from this knowing, not ignoring its wisdom. And that's exactly what we are going to do next.

YOUR AWARENESS IS INSIDE OUT

'There is a voice that doesn't use words. Listen.'
– Rumi

After years of focusing your attention on others, it's a wild ride to turn your awareness back around on yourself. Consider this your tough love lesson number two.

Developing awareness helps us to understand and listen to our mind and bodies, sharpening our senses to become aware of what is occurring within and around us, in real time. Many of us jump into responsibility mode far too easily, running around in circles for other people instead of taking a moment for ourselves. When we do this, we are constantly missing those nudges, niggles, reactions and warning bells.

In order to cultivate self-awareness, we must practise observing singular moments and staying present in order to notice what is going on. It takes practice, that is for sure. It's like catching ourselves out, discovering what triggers us, and making a game out of 'what else can we discover about ourselves today?'. For me, I explored many tools to strengthen my awareness, like walking in nature, meditation, journaling, yoga, breathwork, swimming or enjoying a sunset.

Yet the most powerful practice has been establishing five-minutes of mindfulness.

Like everything, it comes with a warning – every day will be different and what matters is that you turn up for it. Doing it is better than not, and perfection doesn't matter. A practice is a daily dedication. There have been times I've started and not got through it, but I gave myself the space to at least explore it. There was a day a few weeks back when I could not sit still. I got through about three minutes, and my body started screaming, I was wiggling around and my head felt wired. I discovered I was agitated. Didn't exactly work out why. But over my years of practice, I have learned that it provides me with the knowledge of how to deal with what's coming up. When this feeling has been present before, I know that I need to calm my nervous system. Usually because I am on the brink of stress.

Other days I sail through the process, and finish with a sense of peace. I would love for you to try it and see what you discover about yourself.

FIVE-MINUTES OF MINDFULNESS

The art of mindfulness is about observing yourself. It requires us to take time for ourselves. In our fast-paced world, it might feel greedy, but the reward is truly worth it.

The aim is to deepen your knowledge of your mind and your body – physical sensations, emotions, and energy.

How To Do It:

7. Find a super comfy spot to sit. It can be a couch, a pillow on a yoga mat, a rock by a river or even your bed.

SHIFTING YOUR FOCUS

2. Clear all distractions – no music, no kids, no one walking in – that includes your pets. You are taking a moment for yourself.
3. Take a breath – you will perhaps have been rushing to set this up. So take a big breath through your nose. Feel your belly expand. At this point I like to sigh to release whatever tension I'm holding.
4. Settle yourself into your seat. Have another wiggle if you need.
5. Set a timer – phone or watch for five minutes. Put that device out of sight but in reach to turn off once complete.
6. Hit start.
7. Breathe and observe your surroundings, observe yourself.
8. Allow thoughts to pass through you; accept them and allow them to go on their way and don't follow them.
9. Address your body and what it might be saying; adjust your posture; take a breath again.
10. Breathe, slow it down. Surrender to your own comfort or discomfort.
11. We are staying in the moment until the timer goes off.
12. Timer sounds, you are free to sit a little longer, or open your journal and answer the following questions:
    - *What happened in my body during my practice? Any physical sensations, aches, pains, tingles?*

- *Were any of my other senses triggered? What did I see, hear, taste, smell, touch?*
- *Were there any emotions present? If so, what where they? How did I become aware of them?*
- *Were there any moments that pulled me? If so, what were they and what did they mean?*
- *What thoughts were playing out during my practice? Which ones were the most repetitive? Which ones surprised you?*

Write down any other observations from your five minutes.

What is so powerful about this practice is that it gives us the opportunity to learn more about ourselves. From days when the rushing consumed us, to negative thinking loops, to an ache in our body. We can discover so much when we take the time to actually observe. Sitting with ourselves can be hard at first, but start small – five minutes. You can look around the room, you can tap your finger on your leg if you need; the aim is to become comfortable in your own skin. Capable of being in your own skin. Confident that you are exactly where you are meant to be.

In the next chapter we are going to go one step further with our bodies and learn more about our emotions and how to deal with the big ones that arise. It's about becoming comfortable with the feelings that most of us want to run from, so we talk through how to move them with grace.

Chapter Three

RELEASING & LETTING GO

SUMMER AFTERNOONS IN OUR RAINFOREST house would test the limits of anyone. The air thick with humidity, not even a waft of a sea breeze through the trees, the sun blazing like an oven with the door open.

Gathering all of my strength, I would peel myself off the couch, while the kids watched *Play School*, their thirty-minute slot of TV time. Left to my own devices, I could have gone to the toilet uninterrupted, but I chose to start dinner.

One particular afternoon, the motherload of what I was carrying on my shoulders was so heavy, nothing was going to pull me out of the spiral of doom that consumed me. Life was wearing me down. Having two kids under the age of five was like riding a rollercoaster over and over again, with small moments of pause, but not enough to reset. Each day felt like a push, which only reminded me of how much of a failure I was. Nothing was easy. Nothing was working. My husband was preparing for his next three-week shutdown at work, so he was out of the house for sixteen-plus hours every day, leaving me to pick up the house and parenting load.

I was a mess.

My stomach was in knots, while my heart raced, and the thoughts inside my head were running on a continuous hamster wheel. I suppressed it all. I was surviving. I had a family to look after, and a husband I didn't want to let down again. I didn't want my friends or family to see that I was being pulled into the dark.

Standing in the kitchen wielding a knife, holding all of that in after another let-down at work, I fought back tears. I turned the music up in a war against the children's blaring TV. There was stuff everywhere. From the front door to the bedrooms, I even had to kick plastic toys out of the way while I attacked the vegetables with rage.

Today it felt like a chore. I felt steeped in pressure that was increased by two 'starving' children, despite having a snack thirty minutes ago. The constant nagging added a heightened sense of urgency to the situation. I somehow turned into a crazy lady who just needed to get the job done as quickly as physically possible.

My husband strolled through the double doors on his way to the fridge. I swallowed the rock in my throat, feeling its every move as it made its way down. I saw his face questioning what the hell was going on. The tears wanted to remind me that they were still there. I fought back; my body was getting prickly and hot. Looking down, focused on the task, I knew he was there. I didn't want him to see me.

Every day, without fail, when he arrived home from work, he asked me how my day was. Today, I got a concerned, 'Are you okay?'

Fucking busted!

There was absolutely nowhere to hide. I was cornered in the kitchen; the heat was unbearable.

I quickly threw an unconvincing 'yep' back at him and continued chopping away, pushing down the anger that I felt in that moment. Those poor vegetables really copped it, as I hacked my knife through them. Roy moved closer to me.

What the fuck is he doing? Can't he see I'm making fucking dinner? I had tunnel vision of the task at hand, and that was all I could cope with in that moment.

He moved into my space. *What the fuck does he want?* I was trying to cook dinner! His children were starving – though I had no clue where they'd actually gone.

Leaning in, he gave me a kiss, but it only made me tighten up. My head at that moment was filled with 101 things I needed to be doing.

'What's wrong?' Bless his heart. My man is honestly the kindest human I know, but what happened next, I don't think he was ready for.

Throwing my knife down onto the bench, making sure it made a noise, I moved back a couple of feet to get some composure. It felt like he was threatening me by being in my space and asking me what was wrong. *Well, where do I fucking start?*

The next two minutes, I tried to hold my emotions back, fighting them, as words flew out of my mouth, tarred with frustration, tears welling up. 'I've got so much to do and I don't know why it's not working. I don't get it! I feel like I am the one that has to do everything. I'm tired, exhausted, the kids are wild and honestly, I really don't give a shit anymore.' The floodgates were opening as I fought, and blamed, and made excuses, and swore. Finally, I ended with, 'I give up.'

He tried to give me a hug. I was raging and pushed him away. He pulled me closer, and I broke.

I blubbered, tears rolling down my face while the snot joined the party, soaking his shirt in the process. I felt so helpless, like I was carrying the weight of the world on my shoulders. I couldn't see a way out.

I had been holding all of the world's problems in, made them mine, and now they had got the better of me. *Total bastards!*

REACTING VS RESPONDING

That explosion of emotions came out of nowhere, a total overreaction. Our mind likes to keep us safe, with patterns based on survival, operating on autopilot. Emotions, given the opportunity, can overrule logic, taking action without thinking about consequences.

The majority of us live in 'fight or flight' mode, on edge and clinging desperately as we go from one thing to another, in order to survive and meet our basic needs. So when we feel under attack, we react. Instead of observing what is going on within ourselves, we are continually brushing aside what we feel or notice in our bodies. Our unconscious mind triggers stored emotions, and we let rip. We feel it rise, but often can't put words to those emotions.

REACTING:

Trigger → ~~Emotional reaction~~ = Our normal behaviour

By exploring the root cause of why we react, now we can learn how to cultivate new responses. Instead of instantly saying yes to a party we don't want to go to, or lashing out after someone provokes us, we can learn to take a moment to tune in and listen to our body's wisdom.

In order to start responding better in situations, we must learn to pause. It really is that simple.

RESPONDING:

Trigger → Pause: Self check-in → Pull: Inner resources → Response = A better way of living

When we feel the rise of emotions, it's time to take a few breaths. Observe. Yes, we have all the feels right now. Ask yourself:

- *What is happening within my body?*
- *Do I want to run and hide?*
- *What are the emotions that are coming through?*
- *What is happening to my energy?*
- *What is causing me to react this way?*

From here we can tap into our inner resources, in the pause, to explore our body's response. This gives us information to help us to understand the big emotion we are feeling, and to find a better way to respond.

Children react when they don't get what they want; it's called a tantrum. Yet when an adult reacts with an outburst of emotion, it comes from a long-standing pattern they have created. As adults, many of us don't want to take responsibility for these behaviours, and we find it easier to blame things around us. Or we suppress all the big feelings and push them so far down that we pretend they don't exist, for fear of having an emotional outburst. The shame it carries is heavy.

Reactions are formed by patterns. Breaking the pattern requires us to stop, take a breath, and figure out our best response from the knowledge we already hold, in order to honour our truth.

Often these moments happen so quickly that we can find it difficult to bring everything together fast enough. It does come with practice, and developing a healthy response is a muscle that we can build over time. Until then, we can buy ourselves a moment to create a plan of action. When presented with a situation that makes us want to react, it's okay to take time to process, to circle back and to finish the discussion.

This allows us time to consider the best course so that we can have accountability for our actions. It's important to acknowledge that we will come back with an answer, instead of leaving the other person hanging. No one likes a person who always bails just as the party is about to begin, with some crazy excuse as to why they are not there. Follow through! Take ownership of your voice.

MOVING THROUGH EMOTIONS

When Roy held me through the meltdown, I felt my body relax, surrender, and lighten. It wasn't easy, it felt unfamiliar, and looking back it makes me sad that I haven't always felt safe to express myself and share what was going on.

This moment in our relationship was a huge turning point. The man I loved was standing there in his snot-stained shirt, giving me the opportunity to lay the cards on the table and say it all. He patiently held space for me to be a mess. My delivery was awful. His presence was a revelation.

Like many mothers, I had a different standard for how I treated my kids, and how I expected to be treated. With my kids, when the crazy wild emotions came to town, we rode the wave together, and helped them pass – judgement free. There was no 'You're all right, pick yourself up,' after someone has just fallen in tears, no 'You'll be okay, there's no need to cry,' or 'What are you crying about? It's just a scratch.'

I had never experienced what it was like to feel safe enough to show others when I am upset.

Big emotions like sadness, grief, anger and frustration have a lot of shame attached to them. Society doesn't want us in that space; it doesn't know how to handle it – we should be happy all the *fucking* time.

Life doesn't work that way.

But guess what! We are here to experience life, all of life, and it ain't roses all the time. I'm a big believer in giving ourselves a grace period when we need one. There are times when we need to process those big emotions. It takes time, especially if we have never let them come to the surface before. It can be scary, the biggest ugly cry is just that – it's guttural, snot-filled, sobbing, foetal position-worthy. To give yourself that moment you are saying to yourself, and to your body, it's okay to feel this way, you are allowed. And that is fucking power.

Moving through emotions helps us to release them through our bodies. We need to do this because our emotions carry a frequency, and I will share more on this later. However, when we keep piling one negative experience on top of another, it gets heavy. Carrying that emotional weight is exhausting. We want to encourage those feelings to move through us so we can get on with life.

So here is how we do it.

I'm going to break down anger and frustration for you, because I find that these are the ones we all most want to resist.

Starting with the trigger – we feel a rise of emotion – then our body responds in different ways.

For me, when I get frustrated, I clench my teeth, my hands become fists, I get hot, flustered, and teary, because I don't know what to do with the surge that is coming up from my stomach.

When this happens, give yourself time, as we discussed earlier. Create space so that you don't say something you might regret later (*ah yes, lived that one*).

Try one of the following exercises, to help get the emotions moving through you.

RELEASING & LETTING GO

Moving Through Emotions

Anger And Frustration

- Stand at the bottom of a set of stairs (roughly twenty) and look to the top. I want you to run up them as fast as you can – let out a 'RAAAAA' as you go. Catch your breath at the top. Check in – how do you feel now? If you need to go again, do it.
- Find yourself somewhere in nature, at the top of a hill, by the sea, or at a secret spot in a forest – I want you to scream as loud as you can. If you're not sure about that, you can also yell out a big old 'Fuck you' – it's therapeutic as hell. If you want to take it up a notch, jump around and flick your hands about, channel your inner two-year-old. Get that anger out.
- If that is too far out of your comfort zone, scream into a pillow in the safety of your own home.
- While we are talking pillows, you can also stack them up in front of you as you kneel on the bed and throw a few punches into them to release anger. The thought of throwing punches can feel terrifying, so you can also karate chop with the side of your hand to get you started.

Moving through emotions is all about expressing them through the body, so you are able to feel, see, and hear them. Discover how to move emotions safely – try punching bags, axe throwing (which I've discovered in Scotland), rage rooms where you can go and pay to break stuff – how cool is that? Don't be nervous to explore this side of you – it's okay. And it's okay too if tears come – it's an emotional release.

Sadness and Grief

This list is all about encouraging the tears.
- Watch a sad movie if you have been fighting the tears away.
- Curl up into a ball and surrender to the pain as the tears roll down your cheeks.
- Write a letter to someone or even to yourself.
- Write about what has happened – just put all the thoughts and emotions on paper without hesitation. Nothing is off limits, and you can say whatever you like. You don't need to reread it. Just be comfortable with the words that have moved through you.

Moving sadness and grief requires us to be gentler with ourselves. Sometimes our greatest gift is just letting those tears go, with someone we love, or on our own. Explore different ideas to find what works for you.

Note: Drink extra water whenever big emotions come to town. Think of it as flushing the emotional toilet; you are stirring up what's happening inside, putting fresh life force within.

Journal Prompts:
- What caused this rise of emotion?

- What emotion am I feeling?
- What effect is it having on my mind and body?
- How can I move my body to release the emotion that I am experiencing?
- Who can support me while I give myself the time and space to heal?

SUPPORT SYSTEMS

Roy asked me, 'Is there anything I can do?'

Trying to find a calm moment in the middle of my greatest meltdown, I rattled off, 'I just need to finish dinner, get the kids off to bed, I have loads of work to do, then I need to—'

He interrupted me and said, 'I will do the dishes, and sort the kids tonight, so you can go and do what you need.'

Instantly, I felt a wave of guilt. Now not only was I a sobbing mess, now I was going to abandon my family for the night to be selfish and do something for me! It was like I couldn't win.

Over the following weeks, Roy did the dishes every night while I worked at my laptop. That is what a good support person does. They create space for you while you ride the wave of emotions or challenges that are present in your life.

On this occasion this all worked out but, don't get me wrong, I went about it all the wrong way. I erupted. I left it to the last possible minute, when I just couldn't take it anymore. I believed that I had to handle everything myself, and we will go there in a minute. But I know now that I could have totally handled the situation better, by not letting things build up. I was resentful about everything I was carrying, yet I didn't say so and I rejected any offer of help.

This is where having a support crew in place as we deal with the big stuff in life is helpful. We are more likely to come out the other side faster, with a deep sense of security, feeling loved, cared for, making our healing easier to digest. Don't worry if you can't identify your support crew, we are coming to that next.

In the throes of darkness, we may also want time alone. But what we need to know is that there are people who are ready to catch us. Let me ask you this – if your best friend needed you, would you be there?

Hell yes!

Of course you would, so this is where I'm going to remind you that you have people who are ready to do the same for you.

Ask for support, share what's going on – don't leave it to the last moment hoping it will go away.

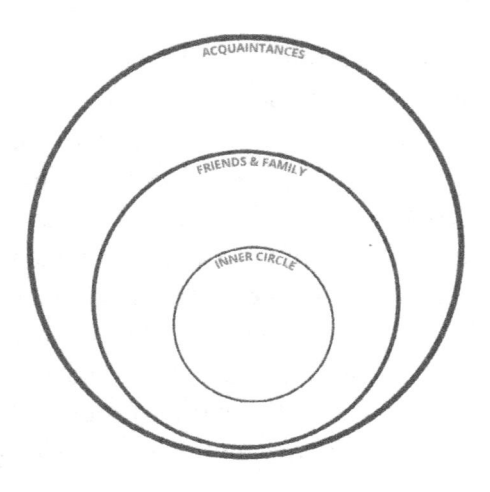

RELEASING & LETTING GO

Building your Support System

INNER CIRCLE: (1–5 people) These are the people who share our secrets. They are the privileged few who have the most in-depth experience of us. They are the ones we love to call to celebrate, or to have a whinge. There is a high level of trust in this relationship.

FRIENDS AND FAMILY: (5–20 people) Think of this as your crew. They are your favourite people to hang out with. The ones we invite over for Friday night wine, midweek pizza or a birthday celebration. We share common ground with them, we find it easy to talk to them, and most importantly, we love to be around them.

ACQUAINTANCES: (10–75 people) These are the people we talk to daily; they can be work colleagues, family members, friends we don't know that well, or beyond. Living in a small town in Australia, we had the vibrant Sue at the post office, Brett at the butcher and Jack at the coffee shop. We used to stop and chat when we were there; however, that was far as our relationship went, it was friendly banter. Our acquaintances don't get a full picture of what is really going on. That is reserved for the two inner circles, which is a privilege.

OUTER SPACE: These people are out of our radar; they hold no significance in our lives. They might be people we walk past every day but haven't built a rapport with.

The great thing about our support system is that we are in control. We know what it takes to become our friend. There is nothing wrong with trying to put someone in one of our circles to see if they make the cut. If they don't, it's all good, put them back where they came from. This exercise also helps us to see which relationships have the most significance in our lives, and who gets our energy.

NOTE: There are no rules as to who goes where in your support system; your numbers may be different to someone else's. This is about identifying the people who are important to us, and the relationships that we value the most.

TAKING RESPONSIBILITY

Imagine me standing at our kitchen bench with my chef's knife in hand, chopping veggies like a woman possessed. Trust me, you wouldn't want to walk in while I'm wielding a sharp knife – I look scary as fuck.

The responsibility I placed on myself to create a wholesome meal for our family was one I took very seriously. It was like a pressure test in the *MasterChef* kitchen, but you only had twenty minutes.

I saw it as my role as a wife, as a mother, as a woman, to feed my family. It was one of the duties that I felt I had no choice in. I'd watched all the women in my life take care of the home, so I just assumed that I had to do it all too. The chores around the house – the dishes, the bathing of the kids, the endless pile of laundry (a.k.a. Mount Washington) – were not my favourite. But I did them because I believed I had to.

What this belief did was rob me of all the joy and creativity that lived inside of me. I was constantly convincing myself that motherhood, and being a wife, was my new life and this was what came with it. The 'okayness' of life was hard to swallow, especially when I was unwilling to admit that it annoyed me.

Each day was an internal battle, because I knew there was more to life than endless housework and toting my kids around. Some people thrive on it. Me, I love my kids, but I see life as an opportunity to be who we are, to live and not be defined by the expectations of others. Fuck perfection, fuck labels, and fuck roles handed down through the generations.

I knew all this, but I still felt guilty when I didn't clean my house before someone came over.

Seriously, why?

I was a total approval addict. I believed it was my responsibility to keep everything running smoothly. Making sure the outside world saw that I had it all together. And for what? To lose my own sanity!

Handing over a basic task to my husband, like washing dishes, was a test of my need to control things.

What are you personally responsible for?

How we interpret responsibility is important. We can either see it as a sense of duty, a moral obligation, or an understanding of how one should behave. Or we can see it as an opportunity to make decisions for ourselves and act according to our truth – this is self-responsibility.

Self-responsibility is power.

F*CK APPROVAL, YOU DON'T NEED IT!

It's acknowledging ourselves first over others, and that there is no need to control or gain approval. That sense of responsibility is what I hope you start to choose for yourself.

We are responsible for our:

Thoughts
Decisions
Behaviours
Actions
Emotions
Reactions
Presence

Journal Prompts:

- Review your daily routine. What tasks or responsibilities are personally yours? Break it down into: home, work, family or other.
- Identify areas of your life where you feel a need for control. Are these areas truly your responsibility, or are you imposing unnecessary expectations on yourself or others?
- Consider the expectations placed on you by society, family, or culture. How has this influenced the way you take responsibility for the above tasks?
- What tasks do you find draining or unfulfilling? Identifying these can help you to get support or outsource.
- Explore the concept of guilt in relation to your responsibilities. Are there specific tasks or duties that trigger guilt when left undone? Why do you think you feel guilty, and is it a rational response?

- Consider the roles you play in your relationships (as a partner, parent, friend, etc.). Are there responsibilities you've taken on that belong to others, or vice versa? What are they?
- Think about a time when you delegated a responsibility to someone else. How did it feel to let go, and what was the outcome? Reflect on the importance of trusting others with tasks.

LETTING GO

Letting go of a task isn't easy.

Letting go of taking responsibility for something isn't easy.

Letting go of pain isn't easy.

Letting go of someone isn't easy

Letting go of how we think our future is supposed to look isn't easy.

For me, releasing and letting go took a journey. It started with me identifying what I was actually responsible for. Then I began to slowly detach myself from what wasn't, including some of my past – the mess, the regrets, and the beliefs.

What I have learnt about letting go is that it takes perseverance.

There is so much outside of my control. I had to focus on unravelling one thing at a time; the process varied from weeks to years. It took a year of actively concentrating on letting go of self-judgement, a few months to surrender to my hubby doing the dishes his way, a week when my daughter decided to take the scissors to her fringe.

Letting go doesn't mean that we lose it forever, it's about making it easier to live with.

Handing over the task of dishwashing meant that I had to address my belief that 'women wash dishes' and all the guilt that I carried. I felt embarrassed about my husband washing dishes instead of me. He was the provider for the family. Washing dishes was my role, my responsibility. The loop goes on.

It wasn't about the dishes.

It was about asking for help, and my belief that 'women wash dishes'.

I didn't want to be seen as weak, not holding up my side of the bargain. The expectations I placed on myself were high. The thought of being seen as a failure scared me, and I didn't want to admit the truth. That is why I had kept it all in in the first place. I was embarrassed. I was scared.

Imagine what people would think!!!!

Feeding my approval addiction was easy. Releasing it took time. I had to take a breath and examine my life, unravelling one story at a time, until I became comfortable with my truth.

Exercise – Let Go, Forgive & Accept:

This practice gives us perspective and insider knowledge about thoughts and emotions. It's about taking ownership and responsibility for our actions, learning from them, and forgiving ourselves.

I've used the following process to help me move through difficult situations, tension and blocks (my own

RELEASING & LETTING GO

thoughts that were stopping me from having the life I wanted – such as 'women have to do the dishes'). I've used it to say goodbye to different chapters of my life, relationships, and past versions of myself.

This exercise is not 'one and done'. It's about repeating it daily, until you can no longer think of any excuses as to why your statement is true. Until there is no longer any emotional baggage attached to it. Let the tears flow, breathe into all the emotions that come, and write them down.

PART ONE

This needs to be your current belief/story – 'It's my fault that I'm (fill in the gap), I need to work hard, I am not enough' etc.

I am letting go of: _____

_____

_____

_____

_____

_____ as it no longer serves me.

PART TWO

This is where I want you to pick the first thing that comes into your head – a situation where the phrase above came into your life.
Write it out, get specific – what happened, who

This behaviour/pattern/story *(pick one)* was created/learned/experienced *(pick one)* from:

_____

_____

_____

_____

_____

_____

_____

_____

_____

F*CK APPROVAL, YOU DON'T NEED IT!

was there, where were you, what did it feel like, what was the triggering moment? Release every moment of how it unfolded. An example: reliving the moment a parent said to you that you are useless and how you believed it, etc.

PART THREE

It's time to take a big picture, look at your story, and face a few home truths. Rewrite these following prompts with your answers.

I forgive myself for believing… *(insert below your belief from part one)*

_____

… and accept that this is a behaviour/ pattern/story *(pick one)* that I have created/ learned *(pick one)* and acknowledge that it no longer serves me.

RELEASING & LETTING GO

List the excuses you made that backed your belief/ story (e.g. that I wasn't smart/ pretty/fast enough, money doesn't grow on trees).

I forgive myself for the excuses I told myself that…

_____
_____
_____
_____
_____
_____
_____
_____
_____
_____
_____
_____
_____

… and acknowledge that they no longer serve me.

It can be hard to admit the truth, this is our opportunity to take ownership of the role we played, we will go deeper on this on the next page.

I forgive *(any/all of the people who came up in the story – list 'em)* for teaching/showing me *(pick one)* this story/behaviour/pattern *(pick one)*.

_____
_____
_____
_____
_____
_____
_____
_____
_____
_____

F*CK APPROVAL, YOU DON'T NEED IT!

PART FOUR

Rewrite this following prompt with your answers.

I am grateful for *(insert anyone/anything that came up in the story)* for teaching/showing *(pick one)* me this lesson because…

_____
_____
_____
_____
_____
_____
_____
_____
_____
_____
_____
_____
_____
_____

What do you know now? Share your discoveries from working through that story and belief.

I am grateful that I have learned that… _____

_____
_____
_____
_____
_____
_____
_____
_____
_____
_____
_____
_____

and I am truly grateful for this gift.

RELEASING & LETTING GO

PART FIVE
Rewrite this following prompt with your answers.

I let go of this story *(insert your story from part one)*. It no longer serves me.

_____
_____
_____
_____
_____
_____
_____
_____
_____
_____

PART SIX

Create an affirmation to finish your release – a new positive statement.

_____
_____
_____
_____
_____
_____
_____
_____
_____
_____
_____
_____
_____
_____

(Write your affirmation 10 times.)

Part Two

START BELIEVING

Chapter Four

CONNECTING TO YOUR BODY'S WISDOM

BELIEVE IT AND...
- ... you'll do it
- ... you'll be it
- ... you'll have it
- ... you'll see it
- ... you'll touch it
- ... you'll feel it

But first you need to get to know it.

Connecting to your body's wisdom is learning self-awareness, self-responsibility, and letting go of control. A process that requires us to trust and feel through all the emotions, in order to develop a deeper understanding of self.

It's all about you. We explore how to connect with and embrace ourselves inside and out, to face our excuses, and get our mind on board, so that we can express ourselves freely. This is permission to experiment, and to stop giving a shit about what other people think.

We need to encourage our mind and body to work together so that we can establish a solid sense of self.

This chapter focuses on our body's whispers, soul murmurings, gut feelings, and spine-tingling goosebumps. We explore the three parts of the self that work together to communicate with us, enabling us to work with our feelings, understand our soul at a deeper level, and see how our physical being is sending us messages. This is our base to learn how to believe and trust ourselves.

Think of your body as a vehicle that moves us around from A to B with an alarm system, and an intuitive GPS. Our body is what people see and feel, and it gives us the opportunity to express ourselves. That alone is powerful.

When I think of the self and all of our capabilities, I am surprised how much wisdom is stored in our body. Our physical body expresses our emotions; our emotional self is how we feel and our soul's vibration is the energetic frequency that others experience.

When I was twenty, I had the crazy idea to travel to the other side of the world, leaving the comfort of what was familiar. I was ticking boxes, and none of them actually made me happy. I was doing what I thought I was supposed to do. Study, get a job, pay the bills, probably meet someone, and get married. The pressure was suffocating. The lead-up to this decision was based on how others talked of travel, their experiences, freedom, plus a boy I kinda fancied.

CONNECTING TO YOUR BODY'S WISDOM

I bought a ticket with a six-week window to get my working visa, and to save as much money as I could to get me there. Three weeks before my arrival, I was ghosted by the boy.

Hurt and fragile, it made my goodbyes even harder.

Boarding the plane with mixed emotions, my reality was becoming apparent, thanks to the choices I had made. Life was a mess, and I was running away from it all. I didn't share my secrets out of shame – the fear of being judged, pulled apart, and that my mental state would be questioned. Severing ancestral ties wasn't something someone does – I know they all expected wild and weird from me, but this – leaving! Even I began to question myself! The tears burned as they rolled down my cheeks. I fought down the terror as I sat in the window seat watching the city get smaller and smaller.

It's too late now. I've got to follow through.

But things did fall into place, I found a two-week yoga residency complete with accommodation in Somerset. This would be where my journey began in the UK. It felt safe to have somewhere to go.

The first few days were spent settling in with my new family. The kids even watched *Neighbours*! They had all the questions about my homeland. Marianne laid out my tasks for the week, and I was surprised at how little I had to do each day.

Too easy!!

I felt eager and ready to dive in, with way too much enthusiasm; I was buzzing.

The girls left for school on Monday morning. I had

ten minutes to drink a cup of herbal tea, before getting on with my to-do list. I was going to get it all done, as quickly as possible, so then I could mooch for the rest of the day.

I asked for the Hoover and Marianne gave me instructions of which rooms to do. Starting with the girls' rooms, my room and the bathroom, then the stairs needed a once-over, before tackling the living areas. The whole job was done in twenty-three minutes.

Bloody lovely!

I was so proud of myself; I was efficient and my attention to detail was great. Twenty minutes felt like a world record for the size of the house.

Packing the Hoover away with an air of smugness, Marianne caught me and asked, 'Do you need any help?' Confused by the question, I boasted about completing the task in a timely manner.

Her reply was, 'You're given ninety minutes for a task, so you do it in that time.'

'Huh?' My facial expression can only be described as puzzled, as I paused before I responded convincingly with, 'Yes, and I've finished it, in twenty-three minutes, that's pretty good.'

'Yes,' said Marianne with a sense of calm, 'however, the yogic way of living is to slow down; think of it as a moving meditation. Have you heard of it? Being conscious of your body and how it moves as you do the task, breathing, observing the mind and its thoughts.'

She had totally lost me. Confused as hell, I nodded and listened. Then, with her encouragement, I set off to hoover the house all over again.

My inner hard-working Australian country girl was screaming inside, *What the actual fuck have I done?*

I've already hoovered, and now I need to do it again, but slower?

It took every ounce of my strength to make this task as slow as possible.

It was excruciating.

I spent the time questioning what kind of a world we would live in if we all took ninety minutes to hoover our houses. Nothing would get done. It's completely crazy; there is too much to do.

I was rushing through life.

What happened next changed everything. I learned so much about myself, and my body.

OUR PHYSICAL BODY

During my moving meditations, I noticed many ways in which my body responded to certain things. I was fascinated by my body's response to slowing down. It took time to understand what was happening.

I did some yawning, let me tell you.

Was I yawning because I was tired? Or because I was unimpressed with the task? Or bored out of my mind?

How our body expresses itself is unique to us. Deciphering the code of what it all means takes time, and curiosity, and we can't compare our body's truth to someone else's.

Frustrated during my tasks, my physical body was processing the discomfort of my limbs tightening, while my blood would burn within me. The loud sighs I unconsciously made disrupted my thoughts, which were left to their own devices in the silence.

Slowing down went against everything I had been taught and believed. It was challenging.

What I didn't know then was that my body was reacting to the situation. My feelings were coming to the surface. I couldn't understand at that moment what was happening, but on reflection it all became clear. I realised that I believed that I was meant to work fast, and that I used this to seek validation.

This is why it is important to enquire into how our bodies communicate with us. There is a reason behind each twinge, niggle, yawn, sigh, or raising of the brow.

When I'm in flight-or-fight mode, I often flutter my eyelashes. It's a nervous reaction to discomfort, a signal that I have lost contact with earth, and become consumed by overthinking, analysing, and questioning my abilities. My senses are on high alert. It's anxiety to the max.

Our physical body expresses our emotions. By learning our body's cues, we open up a relationship like no other. This, in turn, helps us to understand our emotions, and how they communicate with us.

The best way to connect with our physical body is to observe it, through meditation, yoga, being in nature or even journaling. Hey, and if you want to try a moving meditation, try hoovering your house slowly. It's important to remember that slowing down allows us to observe what our body is trying to tell us, and with a little trial and error, we can learn to trust it more.

Journal Prompts to Connect with Your Physical Body:

- Reflect on a recent moment when your body sent you a clear sign, signal or message. Describe the physical sensations and emotions you experienced in that moment. How did you interpret and respond to these signals?
- Think about a recurring physical discomfort or ailment you've been experiencing. What do you think this discomfort might be trying to communicate to you? How can you address or explore the root cause of this discomfort?
- Consider any habitual physical reactions you have in response to stress, anxiety, or other challenging emotions. How do these reactions manifest in your body? What strategies can you implement to better manage and cope with these emotions?

Physical Body Scan Exercise:

Take a moment to tune into your body. Close your eyes, take a few deep breaths, scan your body from head to toe. Notice any areas of tension, relaxation, warmth, or discomfort.

Write down your observations and reflect on what your body might be trying to tell you.

OUR EMOTIONAL SELF

If the physical body expresses the emotion, the emotional self is the house where our feelings live.

While cleaning out the pantry one afternoon, which was already spotless and organised, I struggled with what exactly I was doing.

My emotional self felt frustrated; my physical body felt hot, with a tense jaw, and an unbearable need to sigh loudly.

Unravelling the physical and emotional self can feel daunting and confusing to begin with.

I was scared to admit the internal pain I was causing myself, by pushing down my emotions to conform to society's rules. Like many of us, I was taught to put on a brave face, and to keep my feelings hidden.

I had always come at life at a hundred miles per hour, and being forced to slow down felt almost impossible.

I understood the concept, and I made peace with many of the tasks. And yet, every now and again, a bubbling truth reminded me that this was not who I was, nor was it how I wanted to live.

Approaching our emotions with curiosity and compassion, without rushing to label or suppress them, we create space so that we can own them.

When we challenge the narratives that label emotions 'good' or 'bad,' 'acceptable' or 'unacceptable,' we come to appreciate that all feelings are valid, and worthy of acknowledgment.

Brushing up on our emotional literacy, and building our bank of emotions is a fantastic skill. It's being able to identify, name, and express our feelings with clarity and authenticity. Building a vocabulary of emotions allows us to navigate the nuances of our inner landscape with confidence and fluency.

Instead of 'fine,' are you happy, excited, calm, comfortable, agitated, frustrated, worried, or anxious? *Get to the true meaning of your feelings.*

Our emotional self carries the weight of our wounds and fears. Letting them come to the surface is daunting. Uncovering the truth can feel overwhelming. But it helps us to name it. Then we can take action to help it on its way, as we discussed in the last chapter.

Our emotional self gives us the language to communicate how we truly feel.

The easiest way to connect to our emotional self is through our senses (physical body), with a simple task like drinking our morning cup of tea or coffee.

While you make your brew, look around. What can you see? What does the kitchen smell like? What sounds are happening, in your home or outside? Which cup do you choose? How does it feel in your hands? Now filled with liquid, smell again. Is your cup warm or cold? Have a sip, swooshing the flavours around your mouth. What does it taste like? How does it make you feel?

A cup of tea can either be something we do, or it can be something we experience.

Emotional Self Journal Prompts:

- Reflect on a recent experience or situation that stirred up strong emotions within you. Can you name the emotions? Did you notice any physical sensations or reactions?
- Do you share your feelings with others, or do you find it challenging? What beliefs or pressures influence how you communicate your emotions?
- How comfortable are you with identifying and

naming your emotions? Are there any emotions that you find particularly challenging to acknowledge or express?
- Imagine yourself fully embracing and expressing your emotions, without fear or judgement. What would it look like and how would it feel to share the full spectrum of your feelings?
- Reflect on how you typically respond to uncomfortable or challenging emotions. Do you tend to suppress, avoid, or dismiss these feelings, or do you allow yourself to fully experience and process them? How does your approach to dealing with emotions impact your overall well-being?

NOTE: Keep a journal, and track your emotions, to help build your emotional vocabulary.

THE ENERGETIC SELF

We've all had encounters with people whose energy is larger than life. They have some cosmic energy that pulls the rest of us into their energy field. We don't know why we are attracted to them, but they simply light up the room, and we want to be in their presence.

Our energetic self is our soul's essence, our spirit's vibration, the frequency that we put out into the world. I like to think of it as a magical bubble of light that radiates from inside us. Total hippy talk, but when I experienced how our energy works, thanks to a very tuned-in yoga teacher, it blew my mind.

As I entered the yoga room, Marianne, with her eyes closed, would say, 'Welcome, Lizzie.'

All I could think was, *How does she do it? Does she peek while I'm checking in at the desk?* I tried all sorts of crazy ways to sneak into the room, to see if I could trick her. But for some reason she always knew.

One day I was brave enough to ask her, 'How do you know when I walk in?'

She simply replied, 'I can feel you.' Looking at her quizzically, I wanted more intel, and she went on to say, 'Your energy is much larger than a lot of the women in the room. I can feel it from further away.'

'Holy cow, is that a good thing?' I couldn't sneak up on people, and my energy bubble was big. *How am I going to do life?*

She laughed softly.

The following week she incorporated some energy work into our yoga session. We partnered up, and did Chi Gong together, playing with each other's energy.

Whoa, I thought. *This feels wild.* I was pushing the other person with my life force, even though we were standing a good metre apart. We were invited to see how far apart we could move from one another without losing the energetic connection. Taking one step at a time, slowly, across the room, until the span was over five metres away, my partner could still feel me and my warmth.

This was my energetic field, expanded, and out to play.

Our energetic body is the home of our signature frequency, who we are at our rawest, most honest self, the one with innate understanding, who knows what we need to hear, do, say, and be.

When I discovered the impact of my emotional self, I was led to the work of Dr Masaru Emoto. He studied the composition of water, and how the environment, our thoughts, and emotions affected it. As our bodies are made up of eighty per cent water, I was curious. Dr Emoto's research showed that, when we speak to a cup of water with love and compassion, it forms the most delicate water crystals, yet when we speak negatively, the water doesn't form beautiful patterns.

I wondered if this research applied to people.

We all want to be 'high on life' and feeling our best. To cultivate that state of being, we need to work with our energetic self. When we feel good, we glow, and our energetic frequency is felt by others. Let's get hippy for a moment, and call it our soul's vibration, shall we? Yeah, even my eyes rolled for a moment.

Each emotion holds a different vibrational frequency. Thanks to the work of David R. Hawkins, MD, I came to realise that how I feel is expressed through my energy field, and that this fluctuates with how I am.

Now that I understand that my energetic self can be quickly altered by my emotional state, I am able to keep my eye on how I am feeling. It's easy to get swept up into doom and gloom when my mind talks down to me, leaving me in a big puddle of negative emotions. When this happens, it leaves me feeling small and contracted, with no energy to give.

Our energetic self knows us, and what frequency we

operate best from. It needs to be nurtured, refilled, and cared for. That is why it's important to set boundaries – to protect our energetic self, to avoid clouding it and thereby stopping it from being its best!

When we know our emotions can affect our energetic self, we can make a game of it. On one of those super sluggish mornings, ask, 'How do I want to be feeling right now? What frequency am I currently on? What is impacting my energy? How can I raise my vibration?'

When I need a little pick-me-up, I put on some classic pop tunes and dance around for ten minutes or so. It changes my mood and my frequency for the rest of the day. This works for me, it's part of my personal toolkit, and in the next chapter we will build your Feel-Good Toolkit.

Connecting to our Energetic Self Journal Prompts

- Reflect on a time when you encountered someone whose energy positively impacted you. What was it about their presence that drew you in? How did you feel in their presence, and how did it affect your own energy and mood?
- Exploring your energetic self, what does your energy or vibration feel and look like to you? Do you notice any fluctuations in your energy throughout the day, or in different situations? If so, can you identify what causes this?
- How do different emotions impact your energy levels and vibrational frequency? List and name them along with any physical reactions.

EMBODIED DECISION-MAKING

Understanding the language of our bodies is invaluable and helps us to unlock a deeper connections to our purpose. It serves as a guiding light from within, nudging us towards alignment with our inner wisdom.

Reflect on moments that ignite joy: recollect a memory that warms your heart – a childhood anticipation of the ice-cream truck's melody on a sweltering day. What were the internal or physical sensations? Did you experience tingles, butterflies? These are the whispers of our innermost truths. Feel-good experiences that expand our energy, leaving a feeling of fulfilment.

Confronting low vibrations: recall disappointment, like being denied the coveted ice-cream while others rejoiced. How did your body react to sadness? Explore the physical manifestation; did you experience goosebumps, tears, or a shake in your voice, which signalled discomfort, as you felt yourself shrink?

Listening to our inner voice empowers us to make courageous decisions aligned with our highest good. A structured approach aids in navigating uncertainty:

STEP ONE: Define your query

What is something you need guidance on? This should be a clear question depicting the one thing you've been stuck on for days. Write it down. For example: should we move house right now?

STEP TWO: Outline options

Write down two scenarios for the outcome. What are

CONNECTING TO YOUR BODY'S WISDOM

they? Don't go too deep into foreseeing the future, just know the direct action that you need to take. Be to-the-point and don't attach any unnecessary emotion. For example, scenario A could be: yes, we could live in a town we love but we would have to downsize to a smaller house. Scenario B: no, let's wait for our dream house.

STEP THREE: Find somewhere super comfy to meditate

Get into a relaxed state, allowing three to five minutes to pass before asking yourself your question again. Let it sit there for a moment. Let it float in your awareness.

Now imagine scenario A. Picture it. What would it look like? If you choose this path, what is the response in your body? How does it feel to experience scenario A? Explore the feelings that come up for two to five minutes.

Now go to scenario B and do the same thing. What feelings and sensations come up as you imagine living in scenario B?

STEP FOUR: Observe your body and its reactions

You should be able to come to a clear decision on which path to take that is guided by your heart and deep inner knowing.

With practice and time, building up the muscles required to listen to our intuition will give us a greater understanding of our truth. This process becomes easier the more you do it and the more you trust your body's responses for guidance.

This method cannot be forced. The outcome will be entirely dependent on what is true for you in that moment.

There is no such thing as a wrong choice. Each decision we make is an opportunity to learn more about ourselves, to discover our truth and live authentically.

HONOUR YOUR QUIRKS

Celebrating our quirks happens when we accept our whole self, embracing both our positive and negative sides. The key to success here is awareness, to discover all of our idiosyncrasies – the good, the bad, and the ugly. They all deserve equal attention.

This is an opportunity to get curious and explore ourselves with compassion and understanding. When we know ourselves, we own our habits and quirks, leaving no room to question who we are. Let's explore those now.

Superpowers & Ninja Skills

It's important to acknowledge our strengths and weaknesses, so that we can use them for good. Looking into those deep crevices might scare us at first, but we don't need to let them. In order to heal our souls, we have to get our hands a little dirty. It's all part of taking responsibility for ourselves.

Many of us can rattle off with ease at least ten things about ourselves that we don't like. Hidden in that notable list of all the things wrong with us are our ninja skills.

I've turned being called bossy into being a badass organisation queen.

I've turned my bluntness into my ability to tell the truth and be honest.

I've accepted that my wobbly bits make me a curvy, sexy woman.

I've turned my shit spelling into a career.

I've chosen to celebrate my oversensitivity and see it through the lens that I am intuitive.

Ninja skills hide in our shadows. They are often the things that we most criticise about ourselves, our imperfections, and the things that people point out that make us feel 'less than'.

Whilst helping to clean up after a party, I was drunk, and being my most authentic, potentially obnoxious, self. I was delegating, and pointing out how to do things more efficiently, while I wielded the broom around the hall, sweeping. Strolling into the kitchen, I continued to give out orders, until my mate looked up at me sharply and said, 'Stop being so bossy.'

Those little moments where people call us out are ripe for investigation. Was I actually being bossy? Hell yes, I was. However, with time, I've come to realise that is how people see my badass organisational ninja skills. It's simply me, and one of my many personality traits.

Our ninja skills need a little encouragement. They are desperate to be seen and celebrated. So instead of taking on our flaws as bad, it's up to us to see them through a different lens. To identify a ninja skill, look at how people describe you. Now, how do you describe yourself?

Turn that on its head for a moment and look at the action that is required to make these things possible. Create a new relationship with your discovery: Turn 'bossy' into 'organised', turn 'blunt' into 'honest', turn 'wild' into 'confident'. It all comes down to the words we use, and how we use them.

F*CK APPROVAL, YOU DON'T NEED IT!

I'm not sure why it's so hard for us to see what makes us awesome. All the positive bits get lost in a cloud of negativity. We all have awesome skills and attributes that we should celebrate more, and I consider these to be the strengths that make us unique.

Superpowers are the skills and talents that we can easily identify. They come naturally to us and make us special on the inside and out.

Over the years, people have commented on the way I dress, and my wild hair. Some of the comments were good, but some not so much. It made me question my appearance and why my outfits of choice were a little unusual. Here's the thing, though: I love to express myself through clothing, and wearing something that complements how I feel is really important to me.

Yes, my fashion choices are not always suited to our clean-cut society, but hell, they make me feel good. And my hair, well, I have loads of it, and I'm sure as hell going to flick it around for a few days after it has been freshly washed, flaunting its lusciousness. I know my hair is epic, which is why it's one of my superpowers. It's part of me.

On the inside, I know my brain is next-level magic. Problem-solving gives me a kick, and I find so much satisfaction in working things out. This superpower has always been present, I use it all the time. It was never a ninja skill that crept up on me, but one that I have stood in for years, like my love of being creative.

Let me ask you this: could you write a list of five things you love about yourself? Five about your internal

CONNECTING TO YOUR BODY'S WISDOM

beauty and five external? By the way, this is not here to trigger you. I want to genuinely remind you of how special you are.

Ask yourself these questions:
- *What do I find easy?*
- *What am I good at?*
- *What do people ask me to help with?*
- *What do I love about myself?*
- *What do I love about my body?*

List them, and you will find your superpowers.

Our ninja skills and superpowers are our gifts to the world. To honour them in all of their glory, we need to share them with the world. It takes courage and full self-acceptance to celebrate them daily in our homes, families, at work and with friends. But they deserve to be flaunted.

Exploring our inner workings needs to be done with self-compassion. It involves giving ourselves a little extra love in difficult times, when we feel 'less than'. It's being gentle with ourselves while we navigate life.

Knowing, and owning, all the pieces of ourselves is complex. But the more we own who we are, the more powerful we become.

Living out our days in truth, and prioritising ourselves, stops us from altering our behaviour to suit others. It stops us from questioning who we are and reminds us that we are not here to change others or to please them. It's letting go of negative self-talk, and making the choice to be present and whole.

F*CK APPROVAL, YOU DON'T NEED IT!

Self-Validation List Exercise:

1. Take out a pen and a large piece of paper.
2. Write your name in the centre of it.
3. In one corner write down five things you love about yourself. These can be qualities, ninja skills, super powers or attributes that make you who you are.
4. Next, in another spot, list five things you appreciate about your physical appearance. Focus on aspects of yourself that you genuinely admire, whether it's your smile, your eyes, or your hair.
5. List five accomplishments or achievements you're proud of. These can be big or small, recent or past, professional or personal.
6. List three things you are passionate about, values or principles that are important to you. These could be beliefs you hold dear, issues that matter to you, or qualities you strive to embody in your daily life.
7. Celebrate your quirks – list anything that makes you stand out from everyone else.

Keep your self-validation list somewhere accessible, so that you can see it and revisit it whenever you need a reminder of your worth and uniqueness.

Chapter Five
EMBODIMENT & EXCUSES

DATE NIGHTS IN OUR HOUSE were few and far between for a long time. With young kids at our feet one hundred per cent of the time, all I could think about was escaping them, even if it was just for five minutes of peace. But instead, I used to come up with a thousand reasons why I couldn't leave the house.

We moved to an area where there were hundreds of yoga classes. I was desperate to attend just one of them. After years of not having a regular yoga practice due to endless excuses, blaming where we lived, lack of time, and having a kid, it was finally time I did a little something for me.

It took months of research to find the right class, which turned into a year, and then me giving birth to our second baby. Yeah, I was honestly searching hard. Roy listened to me go on and on for months. Each time I complained about wanting to do yoga again, he would casually say, 'Just find a class and give it a try.'

There was absolutely nothing stopping me.

Except me and my overthinking head.

Finally, I settled on a gentle Yin Yoga class on a Friday. I even spoke to the instructor, to make sure it was on. I dusted off my yoga mat that had been sitting unused in our last two houses, just waiting for me.

I jumped on my bike for the five-minute ride to the studio. I walked through the two yellow doors, to be greeted by a super smiley yoga teacher and two students already lying on the floor. They looked so peaceful, and I wanted that too, as I fumbled around noisily, nervous, and worried about my kids.

Roy has always been perfectly capable of looking after them, but I had tunnel vision. I believed that it was my responsibility to be there for my kids, and I took that role very seriously.

I rolled out my mat and lay down, like the other people. We were still for what felt like a lifetime. I spent it fighting with my mind, trying not to think about what might be happening at home, my to-do list, my kids, the groceries I needed to pick up, my work. Thankfully, we finally got moving and I started to tune into the music. The class was six poses of deep stretching rest, and each one was meant to allow us to surrender in the pose, instead of extending it.

My mind became focused on how to soften my limbs, even in a standing pose that we were to hold for five minutes. My head was dangling down as my bum was in the air. The intrusion of worry about my yoga pants being too thin, and that everyone could see my knickers, was constant. It took every ounce of concentration to not collapse.

EMBODIMENT & EXCUSES

Big belly breaths, in to fill my lungs and out to gently soften.

Ahhh... I was beginning to relax.

The last fifteen minutes of the class were dedicated to a savasana, a deep meditation. The yoga teacher moved around the room slowly visiting each of us. I felt her kneel behind my head, asking if it was okay to proceed. I nodded. She massaged the back of my neck and the base of my skull. Cupping my head with her warm hands and lifting it ever so slightly. Holding the weight of what felt like the world, while I tried not to fight her. A few deep breaths here felt intense as a tear fell down my face. She went on to tilt my head from side to side. The sensation was all too much, and a stream of tears began to fall. Catching my breath, it was as if I had released a lifetime of worry. Gently placing my head back to the ground, she ran both of her hands over to my shoulders, pressing down as if she was pushing me back into the earth.

I had fully surrendered.

It was an hour of pure bliss, and I walked out surprised at my physical and emotional response to the class. My mind allowed me to be in the present moment. The stress and burden I had been carrying was released. It was intense, but I felt at peace. I had literally forgotten that I had to return to my family only minutes later.

That class changed me as a mother, and as a wife.

I went back religiously every week after that. Because I needed, and wanted, that time to hit reset. I was finally doing something for me.

Denying myself a yoga class was the most stupid thing

I had ever done. It still sounds ridiculous to me now. But at the time, I couldn't see any solutions. The excuses I would rattle off:

'If only I had time to go to yoga.'

'If only there was a class that was at the right time.'

'I wish I could still fit into my yoga pants. I will just have to lose a few kilos before I start.'

'I bet there are no yoga teachers that I like here.'

'What if my kids need me? What if they have a meltdown? What if they are hungry? What if something happens?'

Those excuses stopped me from doing something that was good for me, and I began to realise that yoga wasn't the only area of my life in which I had allowed that to happen.

Just like the yoga class, I had spent months on end talking myself out of asking my mother-in-law to watch the kids, so Roy and I could go out for dinner.

'What if she says no?'

'The kids are too little.'

'What if something happens?'

'What if they don't go to sleep?'

'What if they cry the whole time?'

'I'm not sure the kids are ready for this.'

Excuses, excuses.

Sitting down at the little Italian restaurant at the end of our street, Roy and I chose our meals with careful consideration. It was our first meal out together since having Isla. She was eighteen months old, a great sleeper, and we had absolutely nothing to worry about. As soon as I handed over the menu, I picked up my phone to check if everything was okay. Nothing there.

EMBODIMENT & EXCUSES

It had been twelve minutes since we had left our house. I looked up at Roy as I pushed my phone to the side. He was exhausted; his new job was very demanding, with long hours. He was often called in to work in the middle of the night, and he was still finding his feet. He took a sip of his beer and leaned back in his chair. Neither of us had much to say. The first thing I mentioned was Isla.

'I hope she's asleep,' I said. I knew her pattern. I knew she would be fine, but it didn't stop me from worrying.

We had decided to leave for dinner after we put her to bed, knowing that she conked out after her bottle. This would make it easy for my mother-in-law, who just had to sit around the house and make sure no one came in to steal our baby while we were out. She was safe. But what if she woke up, she needed more milk, or decided this was the night she needed walking to sleep? I didn't want my mother-in-law to be put out because Isla was being wild or out of control. Urgh.

Roy shared my concern, but reassured me, only to glaze over and stare out into the street as he drank his beer. It felt like we had nothing to talk about. The last few months were overwhelming. We had just said goodbye to our dream property and moved to the area. I felt completely lost, and the only thing happening in my life was a small bubbly human who I had to entertain daily.

Our meal came out minutes after ordering. We both shovelled it down like we had become accustomed to, thanks to having a small child at the table with us who also needed to be fed and required our assistance. Scraping my plate clean and placing my cutlery on my plate to signal that I was finished, I picked up my phone to check the time. We had finished our meals in record time and were done after only twenty minutes of being there. *What the fuck?*

Now what? I remember thinking. All I wanted to do was go back home and check on Isla. My husband was exhausted and tired and could do with an early night. Our conversation lacked its usual substance, and both of us were searching for something that we could connect on. The quickest meal felt like the longest awkward pause in our relationship to date. It still haunts me, the thought of us at that table. My mother-in-law was surprised to see us walk through the door only forty minutes after we left.

We both reassured each other that we tried to do something for us. But we failed hard at it. It was awkward as fuck.

For me, spending quality time with my man is how I feel connected with him. So, to realise that this had changed since having children was something I was not prepared for. I had put on a 'mum' hat and wore it with pride, sacrificing my own happiness so my children would feel loved, safe and provided for. I took the role way too seriously, and I had lost myself in the process.

Roy and I attempted many more date nights, and eventually we both landed back to a place where we could talk about things other than our kids. It took time. It took us leaning into the awkward mess that was now our life: juggling parenthood, work commitments, and being a partner to the person you love.

We chose us. Our relationship. We faced the excuses we felt about doing it, even when it felt like it wasn't working; we wanted to bring a little magic back into our lives. We needed this.

Not all scenarios have happy endings. There have been times when our excuses have won. The second-guessing, what-ifs, and practical logic makes more sense, stopping us from experiencing what life could be like.

Our excuses are made-up reasons that we create to defend our behaviour, to delay taking action or to dismiss our own responsibility. Excuses want to keep us safe, so the mind sends us on a detour to avoid experiencing something new. It triggers the alert button that makes us second-guess ourselves.

We all make excuses from time to time. Making excuses stems from a fear of failure, being judged and low self-esteem.

It's something we do to allow us to rationalise why we do, or don't do, things.

What's super crazy is when we hear other people rattle off excuses. We sympathise and normalise their explanations, agreeing with what they believe.

Let me ask you this: do your excuses stop you from having the life you want?

ENDING SELF-JUDGEMENT

The reason excuses roll so easily off our tongue is because our Inner Critic is a total bitch. She loves to bring our attention to the pieces of us that are not up to standard. Standing in that yoga class, I was genuinely concerned about my leggings being too thin and my knickers being visible. A total inner-bitch move, to make me doubt myself mid yoga class. I already had so much worry about going back to something I loved after such a long absence. My body was definitely not the same as it was in my twenties. *And who's fault was that?*

It was mine. I was the problem.

Sound familiar?

Intoxicated by my Inner Critic, whose motive was to keep me safe, she made me feel inadequate in more ways than one. The nasty thoughts about how I wasn't meeting my personal standards broke my heart.

What I needed to do was to rewrite the rules and expectations that I had placed on myself. The bar had been set so high that nothing ever felt within my reach. Nor could I accept myself for who I really was.

It's exhausting having to fight your Inner Critic, but trust me, the payoff is great – it's self-belief.

Imagine waking up each morning, feeling complete and led by desire. Knowing that you are capable of conquering what you set out to do. Loving your uniqueness and dressing it up so the whole world can see it. Feeling comfortable in your own skin.

Trusting your ability to make magic in the world.

A place where your energy is felt by the people around you.

Together, we are going to explore your essence, or as my friend calls it Big Deal Energy. We will craft a personalised Feel-Good Toolkit, so you can tap into it whenever you need to. Because it's time to show your Inner Critic who is boss. Fact checking is a great place to start when it comes to negative thinking. But we are going to take that process further and learn how to reframe your thoughts, so that you can get into the energy you need to live your best life.

BELIEF HACKING

Belief hacking is reframing your negative thoughts into positive ones, to evoke feel-good emotions to help us to make the magic happen. This is a step towards learning how to work harmoniously with our mind and body.

In essence it's: Situation → Thoughts → Emotions → Actions = Outcome

Go and get yourself a pen and paper and let's work through this together. Fold your page in half, working on one side from the top to the bottom. Write each section heading followed by your answer to the question associated with it.

I'm going to walk you through how I reframed my Inner Critic's negative voice in relation to that yoga class. Breaking down each section of the process, I will expand on what was happening under the surface for me, as an example.

SITUATION:

The situation is a black-and-white version of what is, or has, happened. It's our current problem that we are wanting to solve. It's what we deeply desire. It's what is sitting in your heart or keeping you awake at night.

When you write down your situation, it's important to write down only the facts that you know about it. All BS needs to be removed along with judgement and emotion.

Question: What is the situation that you are currently working on?

For example, my situation was, *I want to go to a yoga class*. Note its simplicity. Perhaps you are struggling with something; perhaps your boss is being a dickhead; perhaps you want to go on a holiday.

THOUGHTS:

Our thoughts represent the thinking about the situation. It's our internal dialogue, the running commentary that plays over and over again. Here we are making judgements, assuming and telling ourselves all kinds of things. When this happens, it has a profound effect on our body, and on our ability to take action. So, let's explore what your head has to say about the situation, without any hesitation. It's important to be honest here.

Question: What were the thoughts you had during the situation you wrote down?

When I was making excuses, I was thinking, *If only I had time to go to a yoga class. My yoga pants probably don't fit me. I can't start until I lose a few kilos. I bet I won't like the yoga teachers here. What if I go, and then my kids need me. What if they have a meltdown?*

EMOTIONS:

Our body reacts and responds to our perception of a situation. Emotions come through once our story (our beliefs and rules) is confirmed – all it takes is a few repetitive thoughts to make something seem real. Our feelings complement the soundtrack that is playing in our mind and this can be dangerous, especially because our feelings are what drive our ability to take action.

I want you to dig deep here, to be honest about what emotions come up. You are allowed to have any emotional response you want. If you feel anger, that is okay, and if you are frustrated, that is okay too! This is to demonstrate how our thoughts impact how we feel.

Question: How do the thoughts about the situation make you feel?

I like to reread the thoughts I've already written a few times, which gives me an opportunity to explore how they really make me feel.

This is a tool to help you build up your emotional literacy. Being able to articulate how something makes you feel is a real skill. And it's completely okay to have conflicting feelings too; there is a depth to each of us, so acknowledge your truth. Use as many feeling words as you like.

My feelings about going to a yoga class based on what I was saying were: *I felt **stuck**, like it was my **responsibility** as a mother to look after my family, which made me feel **guilty**. I was **frustrated** with myself that I had not kept up my practice. I was **sad** because my body didn't feel like it used to and I was **annoyed** for not living up to my own expectations.*

ACTION:

When we feel good, we take action without even realising; we have the drive to get shit done. When we are telling ourselves all kinds of BS, our body responds and makes us feel like a sack of shit. Thus, the action we often take after this is fairly minimal, right?

I want you to write down what actions you have taken, while the soundtrack played in your head (thoughts above) resulting in all the feelings (emotions above) about the situation. Yes, get honest again, please. It might open your eyes to how you are limiting yourself from moving forward.

Question: What actions did you make/take when you felt the emotions above?

How did those thoughts and feelings you wrote down affect your actions at that moment?

Let's discuss my actions to find a yoga class from a headful of excuses that made me feel anything but great: *I was constantly seeking validation from Roy to go and actually research classes. I was holding in my self-loathing while pretending that everything was fine when it clearly wasn't.*

OUTCOME:

The outcome of our actions can tell us a lot about our mindset, and why we are still in the same situation. When we look at the moving pieces of how our mind and body works, it's pretty clear that we are not reaching our goals because our thoughts aren't on board with our desired destination. It's no wonder we get stuck in never-changing situations.

Question: What is the result of the actions you have taken?

EMBODIMENT & EXCUSES

My result: *I became competent in complaining about not going to yoga, with years of excuses up my sleeve, and all the reasons why it wasn't happening.*

Let's recap how this works so we can re-engineer this.
Here is how it works:

SITUATION = What happened/happening (the facts with no frills)
THOUGHTS = What we tell ourselves about the situation (the inner dialogue)
EMOTIONS = How we feel after listening to those thoughts
ACTIONS = The steps we take when we feel emotions triggered by our thoughts
OUTCOME = The end game, it's the destination after we take action

I bet as you were working through that exercise, you probably noticed how you might have wanted to change the outcome. When we start to look at the actions of what we are doing compared to what we *could* be doing, we know the exercise is leading us in the right direction.

For most of us, taking action is where we fall short. It's so easy to stay comfortable in what is familiar. The unknown lies in our actions, because we don't always know the outcome. We hope for a certain result, but it doesn't always work out that way, so we stop ourselves. When we are in a negative headspace, our feelings match that, so of course, we are not inspired to create change. But tomorrow is a new day!

Now we have an opportunity to review and reflect on what is happening in our life. How our thoughts have clouded our desire, leading our emotions off course, which impacts our ability to move forward in the direction we really want.

REFLECT:

Look at everything you've written down so far, especially your actions and results. Do you think that this was the best course of action for you? What do you think you could have done differently? What would have demonstrated that you had your best interests in mind? What would you have liked to see happen?

Let's turn this around so we can start reconstructing it to make it work for us.

Re-Engineer A Belief

SITUATION: What is the situation you want to focus on?

_____
_____
_____
_____
_____

RESULT: What is the outcome you want or would like to see happen?

_____
_____
_____
_____
_____

EMBODIMENT & EXCUSES

THOUGHTS: Write a list of positive thoughts that you could repeat to assist you in this situation, to cultivate the feeling you need to help you take action. (Example: *I deserve an hour to myself. Yoga is a practice for everyone*)

What do you need to hear or tell yourself in order to reach that result?

_____
_____
_____
_____
_____
_____
_____
_____
_____
_____
_____
_____

FEELINGS: What emotions do they stir in you? (Example: *I am excited, positive and secure.*)

How do you feel when you think about your new thoughts?

_____
_____
_____
_____
_____

ACTIONS: (Example: *book a yoga class, carve out an hour each evening to wind down to support better sleep, hire a babysitter so I can go to yoga each week...*)

Write down a list of actions that you will make towards changing this situation.

_____
_____
_____
_____
_____
_____
_____

When we change our thoughts, it also alters how we feel about ourselves. Just imagine if I had been going to yoga for years, instead of living in a state of being stuck. I would have calmed my anxiety and handled daily life with a lot more grace.

Living in a negative head space is the best way for us to stay where we are. Yet when we feel good, we take action. This could be in the form of play, work, or even helping others. Using this process, we can look at situations with a bird's-eye view, allowing ourselves to course-correct our actions, behaviours and thoughts and in turn stimulate those feel-good emotions.

We all strive to feel good. To be our best selves. That is what our modern society is continually selling us. But in order to cultivate that feeling, we need to focus on what it is that makes us come alive, and bring more of that into our life.

It's time to step into your Fuck-it Era!

EMBODIMENT

It's honestly not just for hippies or the super enlightened – embodiment is embracing who you are, inside out, and living by it. Essentially it's your ability to listen to your senses and emotions, understand your thoughts and beliefs, and trust your inner wisdom.

I had a wonderful astrology teacher who completely poo-pooed psychics, because she believed we all have the answers within us. After years of deep work and exploration, I now believe she was right, hands down. At the time, I didn't understand it fully, because I couldn't make a decision without asking a hundred people what they thought first. But now, I own my desires. Yes, I still love an oracle card to give me confirmation, but not to seek guidance or insight on how my life is going to turn out. Because at the end of the day, I am in control of that. One decision can change everything.

What is important to understand about embodiment is that this is the realm of full self-responsibility and acceptance. I've always described it as my vibe, magic or essence. My friend Leanne calls it her Big Deal Energy. It's where we stop playing small and step into who we really are.

It's about your energy! It's magnetic. When we start stretching ourselves, to be who we truly are, it asks a lot from us, especially as approval-seekers. Every facet of our identity is revealed to the world. And not in the 'I'm naked so I must be embodied' kind of way we see on Instagram.

This is about you turning your light up. Becoming who you have always been. It's living in accordance with your own rules, beliefs and standards. It's living without self-doubt.

No one can take your magic away from you once you own it.

They might try to tear it down, or tear it away from you, but that speaks more to their character than your own. Embodiment takes great courage, plus a lot of experimentation and curiosity, to reveal your essence.

When I first came across embodiment I was doom-scrolling on Instagram, where I was fed loads of images of naked women labelling posts as being fully embodied. I didn't want to get my tits out at the beach at sunset to feel embodied. That didn't make sense to me.

Being challenged on the topic by my friend Michelle, I shared 'Where do these women get off telling me that embodiment requires nudity?' Before long she encouraged me to try walking around naked. I was completely shocked by this suggestion, and responded with an immediate, 'Um, I'm not doing that!'

I made plenty of excuses about why I couldn't do it.

Yet in reality, there were no real logical ones. At the time we lived in the rainforest, and the only thing you could see when you looked out of our house was dense, thick forest. Our neighbours were far away, and if a car drove down the driveway I would hear them coming.

In the end, I promised her I would give it a go. My goal was to comfortably walk from our bathroom up to our bedroom, which was about twenty metres away, nude! Each day after a shower, I would streak through the house as fast as I could because I didn't really want my family to see me. I was fucking naked! I felt vulnerable, and fully exposed. Our small kids shared the shower with us in a small confined space, and they ran around naked all the time, but for me to walk through the house? Nah-ah. That was next-level weird.

Clothes made me feel safe and less vulnerable. I reconfirmed those notions due to the fact that most of the houses I had ever lived in were predominately filled with boys. Naked was not something you could casually do.

The crazy thing was, Roy was comfortable in his skin, completely. He walked around the house nude as if it was totally normal. But for me, being nude in our house was not a thing. Clothes were to be worn. It was naughty to show your skin.

I wanted to show myself I could do this. It took me weeks to feel comfortable walking the full length of our house, but it did get easier with time. I moved slower, and even stopped to talk to the kids one day, which was a huge milestone moment. As awkward as it was for me, to them, I know it was nothing.

After a month, I decided to buy a full-length mirror. I put it at the bottom of the stairs up to our room, so I would have to stroll by it and see myself. I started to use the mirror in the mornings to create wild outfits for the day, because when I felt fabulous, my day usually became fabulous.

I had to take the time to repeat the exercise, allowing myself to feel uncomfortable to get to the point where I was able to reframe my relationship with my body. I had to allow myself space to learn that I was safe in my own skin. It was safe for me to be me.

I'm still a lover of wearing clothes when I leave the house; perhaps that is why we moved to Scotland. It's all about layers.

However, I'm no longer shaming myself about my shape; instead I focus on things that make me feel good. That experience taught me so much more than I had anticipated about embodiment: it's not about being nude, it's about being comfortable in my skin. I had learnt to look at myself in a mirror, and I was loving what I saw.

The coming months saw me look for other

opportunities to express myself. I enlisted my friend Carol to teach me how to use make-up properly, because I was guessing every time I applied it to my face. She taught me the importance of moisturiser at the golden age of thirty-five. Yep, until then, a skin regime was so not my thing. The outfits I chose each morning became more special after I had my ears pierced for the first time that year. My mum said no when I was ten, and It was a rule I was still living by. It had to go. I was desperate to have dangling earrings to add a little bling to my essence.

All these things mattered to me. I had denied them in the past, but now I focused on the feel-goods. Which made me unstoppable, and powerful. And that is why we all deserve to have our own Feel-Good Toolkit.

BUILD YOUR FEEL-GOOD TOOLKIT

There are three parts to the toolkit which are: quick fixes, weekly practices and indulgences.

Once you see yourself as an energetic being, instead of just a physical one, you can see how important your energy is. Choosing to maintain your energy demonstrates that you have a level of self-care, to ensure that you are operating at your best. It's not just moisturiser and dangly earrings that will give you the feel-goods, but practices that fill and maintain the energy you are looking for. Carefully designing your toolkit, you can curate ways to nurture yourself.

Quick Fixes

This is a list of quick fixes for when we get into a funk, need to change our energy fast, or gee ourselves up. These are for getting rid of that stuck or stagnant feeling in order to get out of our heads, and back into our bodies.

Get yourself a Post-it note and write ten ways you can change your energy in ten minutes or less. Ideas: ten big, deep belly breaths, power stance, five minutes' dance party, star jumps, go outside and breathe in some fresh air, watch some comedy and laugh, read a poem, do a meditation, have a cup of tea with no distractions, belt out your favourite song, stretch and move your body, write down your thoughts and clear the mind funk, call your best mate, sun salutations, listen to a podcast, light a candle, smudge the house with sage, clear your space of clutter – throw out a few things.

Weekly Feel-Goods

This is our weekly energy maintenance, to keep our feel-good momentum going. Looking after ourselves is not just for when we are feeling a little 'meh'. This list is to help us to be consistent, and to maintain the vibration that we want.

What we are looking for are two or three weekly things you can do that make you feel good. We are all different so it's about finding the things that you love doing, and working out how to incorporate them into your life. If time is tight, start with one, and add more as you get comfortable doing that one each week.

Ideas: gym workout, women's circle, networking events, therapy sessions, sauna, swimming – ocean or laps in a pool – watching the sunrise/sunset, going to the movies, reading a book, yoga class, walk in nature, sports training or games (football, hockey, netball, lawn bowls), bike riding, dance class, art class, an hour dedicated to being creative, singing/music lessons.

Indulgences

There is absolutely nothing wrong with indulging yourself in life's pleasures. I bet there are things that you secretly wish you were doing, or secretly want. Perhaps one of your friends goes to a spa each month, or you heard Jennifer Anniston gets her hair done in a certain way and you want to try it. This is where we look at creating monthly rituals to indulge ourselves, to be and to feel spoilt, because you totally deserve it!

Pick ONE THING each month, to reward yourself for being awesome, to show yourself how grateful you are for the life you have.

Ideas: get your nails done, go to a concert, go out for a lush dinner with someone special or friends, buy all the fancy cheeses to make an epic cheese board to go with your wine, take a nap, hire someone to clean your house, take an afternoon off and do something fun, have a day at a spa, booking a night away (solo), get your hair done, buy something that makes you feel like a rockstar when you look in the mirror (clothes, shoes, lingerie, jewellery, etc.) attend an event, purchase a course you have been eyeing up, get a massage, have a facial.

Embodiment is embracing your essence while nurturing your energy, without excuses.

Don't let your Inner Critic trick you into doubting yourself. Everything you need to be magical is within you.

Express yourself in a way that makes you happy, and that reflects your personality. Show yourself that you matter.

It's never too late to change. If I can pierce my ears at thirty-five, perhaps you could cut a fringe at fifty, rock a leather jacket at sixty or start wearing lipstick at forty. Find yourself in the small things. Look after that energy centre of yours – give it the fuel to be its best. Start Yin Yoga to ease your stress, start walking each week to calm your nervous system or take that dance class for a good laugh and fun.

Ditch all the excuses and stop worrying about what other people think. It's time to dip your toes in. To be who you were meant to be.

Journal Prompts To Face Self-Doubt:

- *What would my life look like if self-doubt didn't hold me back?*
- *What am I afraid will happen if I fully embrace myself?*
- *What scares me about showing others the real me?*
- *What are my strengths and best qualities?*
- *What do I need more of in my life to feel unstoppable?*

Chapter Six

STOP WORRYING ABOUT WHAT OTHER PEOPLE THINK

I'M NOT GOING TO LIE; it has taken a lot of soul-searching and work to discover who I am. What makes me the rebel, the creative, the sensitive soul, the approval-seeker, and the quirky modern-day hippy who loves drinking tea?

With two hands on the wheel, the engine of our 1970s Valiant Pacer was roaring down the highway, with the window cracked just enough so the wind blew through my hair. I had just left our rainforest home, and my family, for a night away with a group of women for a two-day retreat.

The warm air swirling around me only heightened the feelings of guilt, nerves, and anxiety that I was trying to drown out with the car stereo, which was hanging on by a strand of cable ties. Coincidentally, that was exactly how I felt, as I drove closer and closer to my destination.

The thought of being surrounded by a group of women after years of staying at arm's length was terrifying.

STOP WORRYING ABOUT WHAT OTHER PEOPLE THINK

I couldn't relax; my body was tense, but I tried to fight it, amping myself up with my favourite tunes, and trying not to allow old patterns to rule my time away. The truth was that I had been keeping myself safe after the incident with Stacey and the popcorn a decade earlier.

Pulling into the house, my stomach was filled with butterflies. I swung the car door open, hoping I had parked in the right space, only to catch a glimpse of a shiny silver Subaru pulling up alongside the gate. Someone else had arrived, and I turned and smiled, waving at the woman behind the wheel. Her smile shining back made me feel better instantly. I was in the right spot. I continued to watch her gracefully leap out of her car, with her pearly whites, shiny tanned skin, and her linen dress that barely hid her size-zero body. She was stunning. Somehow, I skipped that we looked nothing alike as we bonded over our excitement for our little getaway together. I had calmed the fuck down, and having someone by my side took the edge off as I entered a new space, having never met any of the other women in person before.

Walking through the large Balinese doors, we were guided to meet the others who were already lazing by the pool, their bikinis rolled for maximum sun on their glistening skin, chatting intimately, and taking selfies with all the giggles. I just stood there awkwardly.

Holy fuck, what the hell am I doing here?

I was nothing like these other women. I was already sweating, I had far too many clothes on, and I couldn't replicate their cutesy 'hellos' and perfectly curated dips of their sunglasses. What the actual fuck. I was standing in a million-dollar house without my babies, and I left them for this? I was so far out of my depth. Who the hell was I to be surrounded by these glamorous Insta-perfect women?

Realising the dress code, I rummaged through my bag hunting for my bikini. With my skin an alarming shade of white, I self-consciously threw on a kaftan, perching myself on the last remaining lounge chair by the pool. But not one of them made an attempt to involve me in their conversations. I didn't know what to do.

I wanted to casually laze by the pool and feel sexy, but I didn't.

I wanted them to like me, but I was also scared that they wouldn't.

I wanted their confidence, but instead, I made excuses for my lack of self-care.

I wanted to have their openness, but I worried what to say every moment.

One of them noticed there was something in the pool splashing around. I decided to look up just in case I could contribute to the conversation. I was so desperate to feel like I belonged even though, in all honesty, I was far from curated.

'Oh, my god, there is something in the pool,' chimed one of them as they remained on their lounge chairs.

Another joined her to point and squeal, 'Oh my god, there it is.'

They all sat there dumbfounded wondering what the hell to do. Me being the country gal that I am, it looked like whatever it was in the pool was having a hard time and wanted out of that toxic chemical water. I got up off my chair to take a closer look.

As I stood by the pool looking at this wet animal swimming for its dear life, I noticed that the others had followed me over, standing close, but still far enough away. 'It's a rat! It's a rat!' screeched one of them.

My knowledge told me it was too big to be a rat, even the gross massive ones that I've seen lurking in our rainforest. This was something else. I rolled up the cotton sleeves of my oversized tunic and knelt next to the pool so I could scoop out this poor little creature with a single deliberate motion. I brought the wet animal next to my body, trying to calm it down as I walked it out of the pool area. I casually strolled towards a bit of the garden that looked rather forested and put it down. Focused on helping the poor little guy, I hadn't noticed the other women gasping in shock and remarking how they would never have done that. Yet here I was, some hippy from the bush who later identified the creature as a bandicoot. They could not believe it.

A minute later they were back in their poolside positions catching the last of the sun as if nothing had happened.

My mind started to question why I was even there. Was it simply to help endangered animals?

I was meant to be reconnecting to myself but also to possibly make new friends and lean into my feminine energy. To be honest, I desperately wanted to be them. I wanted their carefree can't-be-bothered-to-stand-up-and-greet-someone attitude, their fucking living-my-best-life-with-my-ass-out confidence.

Nope, I thought. *I'm a fucking mum.*

The guilt I felt about leaving my babies was unbearable. But the possibility of freedom was here – not quite how I pictured it, but it was in my face. I bet these women got to go to the toilet in peace without having a nagging set of feet following them around reminding them how they were always so hungry. That was my life; that was my reality.

During those twenty-four hours, I guarded myself out of fear. I knew I was different, and I was scared to be me. I wanted to be more like them, and so I did what I thought I should do. You know, authentically expressing myself all the time. (Yes, I'm being sarcastic.) I played down my uniqueness in order to fit in. The weirdo country gal was officially out of her depth.

How the fuck did I end up here?

How did I believe this was something I wanted?

I bought into this wanting a better life, but what I got was knowing I was probably never going to be like them. I was too practical, I wasn't polished in my appearance, and I sure as hell looked a little rough around the edges. I put my people-pleasing skills to good use all to avoid the discomfort I felt about feeling different.

STOP ASSUMING

Assumptions are where we try to predict the future. Just take note of the word 'try' here for a moment. Because the gap between reality and assumption is that we can't guarantee the outcome of any situation.

The way assumption works is that we create a theory that we believe, and live by, from evidence that we have collected in our brains from previous experiences. Thanks to some poisonous words that were said to me a decade earlier, I was paranoid about how I came across, terrified of women because they can knock you down in an instant, and my fear of not belonging, ouch, was real.

When we assume, we are future tripping.

Approval addiction makes us focus on others first, which means we spend a lot of time and energy working out how the people around us operate, so that we can adjust ourselves. This ends today.

Looking back at what we have learned so far, the mind really does have a lot to answer for. So, it's important to remember a few of the tools that we have already discussed, like fact checking in Chapter Two and how to reframe our thoughts (aka belief hacking) in Chapter Five.

When I walked into that lush retreat space, I judged the shit out of those women. It came from a place of deep self-loathing because it was pretty obvious I didn't look like them. Yes, I am also a crap person. BUT... I did that because I assumed that girls like them don't like girls like me – we were from two different worlds. This then of course triggered me and led me to second-guess everything that weekend.

I went on a fact-finding mission to prove to myself and my Inner Critic that the bitch was right. Completely ridiculous that I spent so much of my energy comparing myself in silence. Always searching for words to connect, but I had already put a wall up for protection.

People can feel that wall; I pretended to be quiet and reserved. It was a lie.

F*CK APPROVAL, YOU DON'T NEED IT!

One of the girls had a set of oracle cards out in the morning. I loved a bit of woo-woo. Moving closer in an attempt to join in, I watched as everyone picked a card, all talking over the top of one another. I finally asked if I could pick one as the height of the discoveries died down. The card that I received was the High Priestess, and all of a sudden everyone went quiet. What a way to restart the anxiety! Everyone was looking at me, totally in awe. I've never seen anyone get this card before, blah, blah, blah, the owner of the oracles explained as she turned her back on me.

That was proof enough for me to take a step back, accepting that I didn't belong. This was the kind of stuff the girls would do in high school. And as for Stacey, I can only imagine she would have said, 'Yeah that card was obviously not meant for you.'

My assumptions had me walking around on eggshells with these women.

But how did I know that they didn't like me? I didn't really even give them a chance. I went right into autopilot mode to survive. Because I was triggered. It was uncomfortable, and I was scared of being hurt.

The only person who hurt me over that weekend was my Inner Critic.

She kept me looking for evidence to prove that my initial thought of *I don't belong here* was true.

What I have come to understand and realise about assumption is that there is a level of expectation attached. *When I approach the cool girls they are going to go quiet because they know just as much as I do that I don't belong.* Right? No. Wrong. Total Utter Bullshit.

STOP WORRYING ABOUT WHAT OTHER PEOPLE THINK

Assumptions are dangerous.

Assuming is 'trying' to predict the future (expectation), so that we are ready to handle it.

Here is the thing: assuming fucks up relationships. When two people are both guessing the other person's needs or what they are thinking, they are living in their head. They aren't connected. Far from it.

So, let me ask you this – *How do you know what the other person is thinking?*

You can't mind-read! And neither can I.

Then why do we waste so much time and energy worrying about what other people think? Oh, yes, all the fear. Perhaps it's not belonging, not feeling loved, scared to disappoint, worried that you will be seen as less than you already are. It's soul-destroying.

The worry is real, and it's fuelled by our own lack of self-belief.

Assuming stops us.

Assuming lets self-doubt win.

Assuming is pretending we can read other people's minds.

We will never know what someone else is thinking. EVER!! Unless we ask them. If you notice that someone is upset, do you just do what you think you should do for them? Or do you check in to see what they need?

If we take assumptions out of our relationships, we are giving both parties an equal opportunity to be responsible for themselves. Instead of guessing what the other person is thinking, perhaps you ask them. Instead of worrying that you are going to let someone down, remind yourself whose life you are actually living. Instead of avoiding bringing up a subject because your partner is always so tired and grumpy, you finally say the thing.

Worrying about what other people think is about their actions towards us. Their reaction to our 'what ifs'. Unfortunately, there is only one way to find out what will happen and that is to do the thing. If you are not ready to jump right in, take time to consider what you are most scared of, and any beliefs that sit alongside it.

We need to look at our triggers – for me it was a group of women (ooh, scary) and being made to feel like I'm inferior and pushed out from the group. AKA – I was scared of not belonging because at the root of it I had some major trust issues.

Addressing our fears is an important step in ending our cycle of approval-seeking.

I want you to ask yourself the following questions and spend some time journaling and exploring them.

Journal Prompts

- *What evidence do I have for the assumptions I make about how others perceive me, and is it based on facts or fear?*
- *How has worrying about what others think affected my actions or decisions in the past?*
- *What specific fear or belief lies at the root of my need for approval or acceptance from others?*
- *How would my life change if I stopped trying to predict others' thoughts and reactions?*

- *When I assume someone's reaction, what am I actually doing?*
- *How can I fact-check my thoughts and assumptions before allowing them to influence my behaviour?*
- *In what areas of my life can I begin to let go of the need to control how others perceive me?*
- *Does it matter what other people think?*

Get curious; unlocking your fears will feel scary, thanks to the unknown. But it will help you to see how your approval addiction has stopped you from many things. And remember, you can't read minds, so stop giving your time and energy to worry.

We Can't Control the Weather

The organiser at the retreat had asked a lady called Katie to come and speak to us about connecting to ourselves. She pointed out that, in order to do this, we should explore the depth of our judgements. Katie explained that even the weather could impact our lives when we judged it as either hot or cold. My heart skipped a beat.

The weather?

My body continued to curl up into a ball as my mind started to reflect on how this could be. The fucking weather. By saying it was hot, that was a fucking judgement. Seriously?

It was early November and summer was just around the corner, so I thought, *All right, why the fuck not try this out? Let's let go of all the judgement I hold about the fucking weather.*

F*CK APPROVAL, YOU DON'T NEED IT!

I sounded crazy in my head, and even my sarcasm was sceptical. I remember telling Roy how I was going to test this theory. He chuckled. I think he thought I was crazy too. After years of watching people judge others, and make statements based on what they have declared their truth, the weather seemed a trivial piece to sort out.

Growing up in a rural landscape, the first concern on any farmer's mind is the weather. It becomes the topic of long-winded conversations, and for good reason too. Farmers rely on the weather to deliver rain to grow their crops, and sun to dry out their hay paddocks, yet unpredictable weather causes havoc, like hailstones that can destroy a crop in five minutes. It's absolutely devastating.

When I left home, I took 'How's the weather?' with me. I found it fascinating that something I couldn't control had complete control of me!

Despite living in the subtropics, I ain't no sun-loving babe. My skin is delicate; I blotch, I burn, I sweat, I feel utterly exhausted from the Aussie heat. For years, the thought of a hot summer's day would keep me indoors, only to peel myself up off the couch in a pool of sweat. Days would often peak at 35°C, sticky, hot and humid.

I made up my mind each morning when I looked down at my phone and saw the max temperature for the day. Fuck, it was going to be hot. I was doomed!

I would have a small freak-out assuming the worst before the day even began. *I guess it's going to be another unbearable day, I will most likely be a grumpy bitch by lunchtime, and there is nothing I can do about it but wait for it to be over.*

STOP WORRYING ABOUT WHAT OTHER PEOPLE THINK

I was dragging myself, and everyone around me, down in my battle to escape the environment! I set myself an experiment. In order to let go of judgement about the weather, I needed to practise present-moment observations. So, when I got up, I stopped looking at the weather forecast, and I dressed in something that felt good at that time. I had to let go of any assumptions that I had.

It took some time until I no longer waited with anticipation for the heat to swallow me in its fiery inferno and roast me. I was jumping from moment to moment, changing outfits if need be, making impromptu visits to the creek for a fun swim. I just nodded when others mentioned the weather. 'Yep, it might get hot later,' I agreed, but it wasn't my primary focus. I needed to let it go. I bit my tongue to stop myself from talking about the weather or complaining about the heat. Instead, I had to accept it as it was.

That summer, I realised that I had been stopping myself from enjoying life over the summer months, from long days spent with people I loved, to experiencing all kinds of fun in the water. My skin didn't go blotchy and red like it had done in the past. It turned out, I had created that heat in my body because that is what I told it would happen.

Casting judgement, I learned, is one thing, but to then assume the outcome of that judgement is a recipe for disaster.

When I first considered letting go of judgement, I thought it was to stop making statements about others, such as 'All sales assistants are the same,' 'No one should ever walk around their house naked,' or 'That person is this or that.'

In fact, for me it was how I cast judgement on myself. I was holding myself back because of how I perceived the world around me.

The weather is too hot, so I can't go out today.

My judgement was based on my assumption of how things were going to play out. I was future tripping.

Assumptions are dangerous.

How our mind decides to use the information we collect is really important. Yes, we can cast judgement on anything – call it what it is – but we must process it and check it by our own rule book. Staying in the present moment is crucial for this to happen.

Once I realised I projected my thoughts onto situations, it opened my eyes to the fact that I was wasting my time thinking about all the possibilities way too much. The amount of effort required to problem-solve all the endless questions about how people could react consumed me.

We are responsible for how we react to others and… guess what? Everyone else is responsible for their reactions too. We can't control people or stop them from not liking us. It's just an ugly truth, but if that's the case, you don't want them in your life anyway. There is a whole universe of amazing people who want to be with you. Perhaps go back to Chapter Three and look at your support system. I want to remind you that you are in control of the people in your life. Your inner circle are the ones who are cheering you on constantly. While those acquaintances are out on the periphery for a reason.

My rule is, if you wouldn't invite them over for a night of pizza and wine, why does it matter what they think of you? Yep, it doesn't. They are not your key people.

Breaking free from assumptions and worrying about what other people think, means we can break free from the need to control the outcome. Judgement and expectations are left behind. We can focus our attention on maintaining and curating the people around us who support us, who love us for expressing ourselves fully. Self-doubt is triggered by fear, so get on top of that, and don't fall into autopilot behaviours.

AUTOPILOT

There are many things we do on autopilot, like apologise when we accidentally bump into someone, immediately answer when someone asks, 'How are you?' with, 'Fine thanks,' or saying yes to an invitation because we feel obliged to go.

We might also be on autopilot when we brush our teeth, go through our morning routine or cook our go-to favourite spaghetti bolognese. These autopilot settings can serve us well to get shit done. They require little capacity from our mind space, and we move through them with ease, with no harm done to our psyche.

The autopilot settings that we use to do the dishes each day have been set, so we can forget them, because we don't need to use our mental space to navigate a task that we do repeatedly. However, the autopilot systems that we have learned, or feel like we 'should' be doing, are the ones we need to question. These systems almost feel like natural instinct because over the years we have been collecting information to confirm their validity.

For example, it's polite to apologise. Yes, there is truth in that for sure. But do you do it instinctively? Is it just a reaction that you do, even when it's not your fault? Do you skip answering when someone asks how you are feeling because you don't have time to share or because you feel like it's not that important? Do you believe these are just commonplace practices that we all do, and we just expect other people to do them too?

Autopilot systems can be dangerous, especially if we are skipping through moments that need to be met with care. Keep your dishwashing routine, for sure, but question how you react to certain situations, people, and environments. Our autopilot patterns need to be monitored, and a bit of quality control is needed, because as we grow and evolve, so should the way we behave. A pattern we hold as a five-year-old may not be our truth at thirty-seven, and this could be the key to why we seek approval in the first place.

CALM THE ANXIETY SPIRAL

Assumption, control, expectation, judgement, and functioning on autopilot all live in the mind. When the pressure of life gets the better of us, we feel stressed. When we start future tripping, it leads us toward anxiety. It's a cycle that many of us find uncomfortable because the worry about how it's all going to work out becomes all-consuming. We live in our heads, detaching from our body. Our breathing becomes shallower, while our nervous system is on high alert, looking out for danger (most likely for proof about what is happening in your head). We get defensive, nervous and it causes havoc to your body.

In the last chapter, we built our feel-good toolkit; it has a list of quick fixes to help you get out of a funk. But anxiety requires you to get back into your body, to calm your nervous system, and to let the hyper-vigilance go. What I have found is that anxiety can cripple any of us in a moment. The tools I'm about to share are the same ones I give to my clients in the first session. Most of the clients have a wall up, like I did on that retreat. I felt as if I was in danger and didn't really want to address what was going on deep inside me.

Calming your nervous system can help you to find clarity and peace amid the chaos.

When you find yourself leaning towards an anxiety spiral or worry, I want you to remember to come back to the present moment. Breath is your best friend here.

Learning about your anxiety and its subtleties is equally important to practising the following techniques. Knowing when the techniques are needed is about understanding how your body communicates with you. If anxiety shows up with your heart starting to race, and you feel short of breath, that's your cue to do something about it. Get out of your head, and back into your body. Just remember, your body feeds your brain information, so listen.

Feel free to explore the following techniques; try each of them, and alter them to suit you.

TECHNIQUES TO CALM THE NERVOUS SYSTEM

Legs Up The Wall Pose
(Viparita Karani)

The Legs Up the Wall Pose, also known as Viparita Karani, is a simple yet incredibly rejuvenating yoga posture that holds the power to melt away stress and bring about a sense of relaxation.

I'm starting with this because it's made such a huge difference in my household. During our summer holiday, my son had to get stitches, and hubby put his hand up to be in the room when they did it. Turns out, he went as white as a ghost, and the doctor asked him to do this pose on the hospital floor to help him regulate his nervous system. I've been telling him for years that this pose is great as it helps to reduce stress and calms the mind.

BENEFITS:

- Activates the relaxation response (parasympathetic nervous system) and deactivates the stress response (sympathetic nervous system)
- Helps lower or regulate blood pressure
- Calms the mind (which help to alleviate anxiety symptoms)
- Relaxes the body and mind before bed, and improves sleep
- It improves circulation (both lymphatic and venous)
- Alleviates tension headaches

HOW TO: All you need is a wall, and a yoga mat if you want.

The aim is to wiggle your bum up against the wall with your legs up the wall. Hold the pose for a minimum of three minutes, and I bet your outlook on life will change. For those who suffer from anxiety attacks, this is also a great one to ground yourself if you feel one coming on.

MEDITATION

Don't roll your eyes! I know, loads of people are talking about it, and you know about it, but still you may have not got how this meditation thing works. Let me simplify it.

The reason why meditation is so bloody powerful is that it subconsciously helps you to train your brain. Every time your brain wanders while listening to a guided meditation, you have an opportunity to catch yourself, and bring your attention back to what you are listening to. This builds your awareness muscle. In other words, you can learn to master your thoughts, the ones that send you on anxiety spirals of doom.

There are loads of meditation apps out there but the one that I use and enjoy is *Insight Timer*.

MY NO BS RULES FOR MEDITATION

1. Don't listen to a meditation if the person's voice is making you cringe. Hello, it's not relaxing!
2. Get as comfortable as you can. I'm all for lying down, pillows, blankets, the works. Build a nest.
3. Start small; don't dive right into a twenty-minute meditation. Start at about five to ten minutes. This gives you time to build up and get used to doing it.
4. Find a time and stick to it. I suggest most people do

it either as the last thing they do before bed or first thing when they wake up in bed. Yeah, I'm talking already lying down, no need for anything fancy.
5. It's a practice; your mind is going to wander. It's totally okay and all you need to remember is to bring your attention back to what the person is saying.

BOX BREATHING

Box breathing is a breathing technique that I teach to all my clients who suffer from anxiety, because it can be done on the spot, and no one will know you are doing it. And if you want privacy, take yourself outside, or off to the loo for a few minutes.

The reason why I love box breathing so much is it reconnects us to our body when our mind is racing. Plus, it's a trick to distract your mind as you count to four over and over again, which calms your nervous system, and decreases stress in your body.

Did you know that in the UK paramedics are taught this breath to help support them in stressful situations?

BENEFITS:

- Reduces cortisol (stress hormone) levels and may lower blood pressure.
- Helps you to sleep when you are having insomnia.
- Helps to control hyperventilation as you can instruct your lungs to breathe rhythmically.
- Refocuses you when you are having a busy or stressful day.
- Eases panic and worry.

- Keeps you calm while preparing for the day.
- Parasympathetic activation: in response to stress, the sympathetic nervous system triggers 'fight or flight'. Box breathing shifts you to the parasympathetic system, promoting rest and balance.

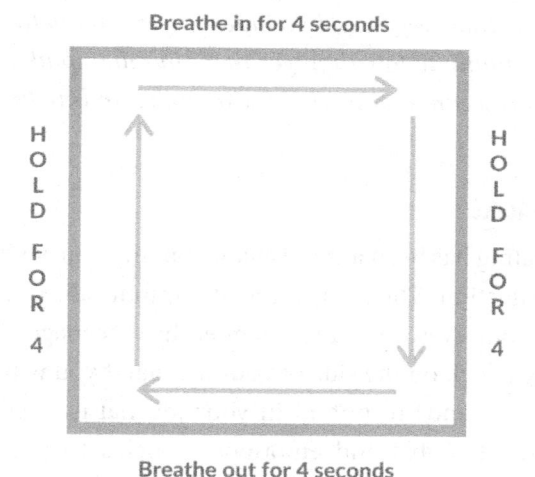

```
              Breathe in for 4 seconds
         ┌─────────────────→─────────┐
         │                           │
    H    │                           │    H
    O    ↑                           ↓    O
    L    │                           │    L
    D    │                           │    D
    F    │                           │    F
    O    │                           │    O
    R    │                           │    R
    4    │                           │    4
         └─────────←─────────────────┘
              Breathe out for 4 seconds
```

HOW IT WORKS:

- *Inhale (4 counts)*: Breathe deeply through your nose and feel your lungs expand.
- *Hold (4 counts)*: At the peak of your inhale, pause for a gentle moment. Allow yourself to be still.
- *Exhale (4 counts)*: Release the breath through your nose and release any tension in the body.
- *Hold (4 counts)*: Once again, hold your breath. Embrace the emptiness with a sense of serene anticipation.

The reason why this works so well for anxious folks is because most of the time we are only breathing into the chest, not all the way down into the abdomen. Repeat this for a minimum of four rounds.

PRO TIP: *For those that fidget. Use your hands to keep count by touching thumb to index finger, thumb to middle finger, thumb to fourth finger then thumb to pinky as you count. You can do this with one or both hands to the count of four.*

JOURNALING

Journaling has been a game changer in my journey toward self-reflection. The great thing about journaling is that it is for your eyes only. Yes, channel those teenage years of having a lock on the side of your journal if you will.

What tends to unfold in your journal is a reflection of your thoughts and emotions. It helps to put things into perspective and also gives clarity. It's a process of self-expression that can bring solace, insight, and empowerment.

There's no right or wrong way to journal. Find a style that resonates with you and dedicate five to ten minutes a day. You can choose from:
- Free Writing: Let your thoughts and emotions flow onto the page without constraint or judgment. I like to focus on the day or the issue that is causing you discomfort.
- Prompted Writing: Use thought-provoking prompts to guide your reflections.

- Gratitude Journaling: Focus on the positive aspects of your life.

BENEFITS:

- A space to release pent-up emotions.
- Putting thoughts onto paper can help you to process stressors, reducing their hold on your mind.
- Improves self-reflection as you gain insight into your thought patterns, behaviours, and desires.
- Improves problem-solving as you write about challenges, analyse situations, and brainstorm solutions.
- Tracks progress as you document your journey, creating a roadmap of your experiences and growth.

NATURE

Nature has an incredible ability to calm the mind and soothe the nervous system. The sights, sounds, and smells of nature engage our senses in a way that urban environments often cannot, providing a refreshing escape from the constant stimulation of modern life. Research indicates that even short periods spent in nature can lower cortisol levels, reduce blood pressure, and improve mood and cognitive function.

One particularly effective practice is Japanese forest bathing, or 'Shinrin-yoku'. This involves immersing oneself in a forest environment, engaging all five senses to connect deeply with nature. The practice encourages mindfulness and presence, allowing individuals to slow down, breathe deeply, and experience the tranquillity of the natural world. Forest bathing has been associated with numerous health benefits, including enhanced immune function, and reduced symptoms of anxiety and depression.

The key to stopping worrying about what other people think is to remind yourself that you are in charge of your own life. Stop assuming, and get out of your head. The magic lies within your body. When it's calm and centred, you can focus on your needs over others. It's a practice, and I'm sure you are starting to get the hang of it.

Chapter Seven
PERMISSION TO GET IT WRONG

AFTER HIGH SCHOOL, I WAS lucky enough to go to art school. It wasn't the exact course I had wanted but I was *in*. I loved drawing, and I really wanted to do art for a living. My spare time at home was spent drawing and painting from magazine clippings, photos, and video clips like 'Do the Evolution' by Pearl Jam. I could draw what I saw, and though my style was a little messy and far from perfect – not like those gifted humans who paint as if it's a photo – my pictures were full of texture, still in proportion, but with their own thing going on.

Each week was packed with practical learning experiences, which I loved. They were fun, and I got to keep my hands busy creating. However, every Friday was theory, and that scared the shit out of me. I loved the learning element, but I bombed the assignments because I had no clue how to write fancy university papers with proper referencing.

My favourite part of the week was my still-life class. The teacher would set up cool installations of plants, flowers, vases, bones, and all sorts for us to draw. We had to use charcoal, not pencil, on butcher's paper. The longer sessions had fancier paper. I never knew how expensive art could be, but buying the paper alone would break my bank at twenty dollars for one sheet. I was still learning, and I didn't understand why I would even want to use a piece of paper like that.

One week, our teacher asked us to bring in a specific set of paints, and we had to mix up our very own charcoal colour. It sounds easy, but take out the black, and I would like to see you give it a try. All you have to use is red, yellow, blue, and white. Good luck.

At first, we just packed up our belongings and waltzed out of the class when it was over. No one saw our work. Then we started to get assignments and we were expected to present them to the class to be critiqued. Eek!

Here I was, a small-town girl, totally out of my depth, standing at the back of the room, and hiding behind my fellow artists as they shared their work one at a time. I watched them as they each spoke confidently about their pieces, each receiving feedback that seemed to me like a standing ovation. I was dreading the moment the teacher called my name.

'Elizabeth.'

I felt sick instantly, as if I was in trouble. I navigated through the maze of classmates, weaving my way to the front. Placing my canvas on the easel, my voice was quiet, and I didn't look up as I explained my painting of five bulldozers. It was my environmental piece about how our world was being destroyed. To be honest, it was not my finest work. I'd thrown it together in a day with the deadline looming. Inside, I knew it wasn't great, and I was embarrassed that I had to show it, because I was not proud of it. I had shown my flatmate that morning and he pointed out that the proportions were all wrong.

There were thirty sets of eyes staring at me. My shoulders began to tense as I waited in silence for feedback. A few people asked questions and, clammy and fighting my discomfort, I answered them, waiting with dread for the all-important moment the teacher signalled for the class to let rip.

Someone called out that they didn't understand it. Another liked my use of colour and texture in the background, but felt everything else was out of proportion. The comments kept coming.

'It has no feeling to it.'

'What were you trying to communicate with us?'

They said all the things I knew but was so scared to hear.

At seventeen years old, it was one of the most excruciating experiences I had ever endured. I was blatantly criticised by my whole class, and I stood there fighting back the tears and terror. They didn't like it. No one had told me that critiquing was a part of the art world. Couldn't we just create art because we loved it?

Discovering that I could put a message into each painting was new to me. I was so used to just drawing what I saw in black and white. The thought that I could infuse something deeper was a little exciting. The only problem was that my imagination would come up with these great concepts, but I didn't know how to execute them. I could work out how they looked in my mind, but I didn't know how to draw them without seeing them already on paper or in the flesh. Visually, there was something missing.

As time went on, the classes became more challenging. Our assignments were about ourselves, and it was really hard for me to navigate that space. I hadn't thought of myself as a conduit for a message. I was barely eighteen and was just creating art because I loved how it made me feel.

Our second semester of life drawing got really interesting, when we started on nudes. My conservative, don't-show-anyone-your-skin self wasn't quite prepared for what was to come. The day came for our first session. I set up my easel with butcher's paper, and had my charcoal ready. A small woman in a kimono walked up to the plinth in the centre of the room, and then suddenly she was naked. I was flustered and didn't have enough time to think about what was really going on. I was trying to play it cool.

I had somehow put myself in this situation. This was about becoming an artist, and all the greats did nudes at some point in their careers, right? But she was naked. I was clothed. There were thirty sets of eyes on her, and she was okay with it. I was still in shock that this was happening. I admired her courage, but I secretly wanted to run out the door.

The models were all different shapes, sizes, and ages of women, who gracefully stepped onto the plinth each week. And then, BAM, out of nowhere, we had a male model. Just when I thought I had finally come around to this whole nude thing. I had started to feel their liberation of being able to pose nude in front of an audience and then swan around in their robe looking at the art afterwards. But this week we had a man sitting in the centre waiting for us as we filed into the room!

He took it all off. The robe was down. My eyes looked everywhere around the room but where they needed to be. Luckily, we were starting with some very quick sketches that were thirty seconds each. Each pose was dynamic in strength; there was something very different about what was occurring, and he held each complex pose for longer periods of time, up to five minutes. It wasn't until he reclined back on the plinth that we were in for a twenty-minute pose. The only problem was that I had front-row seats to a full-frontal that I had not signed up for. For goodness' sake, I needed to grow the fuck up! I was an art student, not a schoolgirl anymore!

As uncomfortable as it was, I got through that class unscathed. I had dropped my judgement around nudity. I got okay with seeing a penis in front of me. Like, really seeing it. Life drawing requires capturing the complexities of the whole body. The next time the teacher decided that it was time for another critique of our work, all I could think was, *I hope that I drew a penis.*

It wasn't the last penis I had to draw.

I went from being a very conservative country girl to

someone who was comfortable with people being naked in front of them. It was a huge deal. I had accepted that in order to change my life I had to get confident with what it was to be an artist. I too had to reveal who I was. If the models could rock their curves, wrinkles and hair, I should be able to do the same.

Our most uncomfortable times are here to teach us things. Hindsight is a complete bitch, let me tell you, as someone who has hit rewind on her many learnings. Moments have meaning.

Over the course of a year, I learned that there is always room for improvement. Those art critics that I survived were not there to shame me but to open my eyes. To improve my work, I could take on their feedback or leave it at the door, depending on which I saw fit. It was about having the strength to stand by my work and own it. Honestly, it takes a lot of courage to show your work, and I've learned the difference between work that I am proud of, and that which I have rushed or am not connected with.

It was a year of experimentation in many ways. My self-doubt rode a rollercoaster most days, not knowing what would come at me next. That first year of living away from home and being at art school was life-changing, and I am grateful for all that it taught me. The way in which I see the world, the way I can still draw and paint, and the way that I understand that not everyone is going to like what I do, and that is totally okay.

Here's the thing – I didn't like all the art of others, either. So why did they have to like mine?

PERMISSION TO GET IT WRONG

Well, because I'm an approval addict who needed validation to know that I got it right.

This chapter is about learning to embrace our mistakes, and that it's okay to get it wrong. This is about traversing the great unknown. Once you decide what you want for your life, the next steps are about making it happen, and most of us jump right into the how. Then usually the mind jumps in with all the reasons you can't.

And perhaps like me you are also scared to fail.

Approval seekers don't fail; we win, we strive to succeed, because failure is our arch nemesis. We have learnt that, when we fail, bad things happen, right? We might let someone down, we might disappoint them, we might feel guilty for our team. Failure is not an option, because it's uncomfortable.

Here is what most people don't know – through failure we learn. I watched something that popped up on Facebook a few weeks ago. It was Owen Wilson, talking about how he wished he had failed more when he was younger. It hit a chord – yes, why did we play safe for so long?

It's because it's the unknown – the scary place that somehow resembles Mordor from *Lord of the Rings*.

But it's not.

Do you remember when you were a kid, wishing life would hurry up so you could be an adult, with all that freedom and independence? That was me. I finished high school, and I was out of there. I got a job, a place to stay in art school, and I struggled like I had never done before. But I did it. I made it through, I paid my bills, I studied, I did what grown-ups did. Because it turns out that was the reality of it. But I had to learn that too. I knew I had to do the shopping to feed myself, and I had to pay rent.

This learning hasn't stopped yet. I had no clue then, and I still haven't worked it all out now. It's ongoing.

The best way to learn is through lived experience.

When you put yourself through an experience, you gain information by doing, your body feels it, and that triggers emotions, and your brain takes on all this new stimulus. Yet when you sit on the sidelines waiting... what happens?

Nothing. You get absolutely bogged down in your head, trying to work it out. And there is a time and place to work things out, but you still need to dip your toes in, to understand the whole situation. Plus, I want to give you a little 'heads up'.

You are in the driver's seat.

What that means is that you have the ability to make choices. Over and over again. Which means that if you make a choice and it's not working out how you want, you have the choice to let it go, keep going, or scale it back. It's up to you.

You've got all the power.

WRITE YOUR PERMISSION SLIP

1. **Grab a Blank Sheet of Paper**
2. **Reflect on a Desire or Goal:** What is something that you want? Sit with that for a moment and ponder what's something you want to try but haven't yet, due to fear of failure, uncertainty, or feeling like you need to have everything figured

out first. It could be related to work, creativity, relationships, or even a personal challenge you've been thinking about.

3. **Write Down What You Want to Experiment With:** Write down the activity, goal, or desire, be specific. For example:
   - 'I want to start writing my novel.'
   - 'I want to try painting for fun.'
   - 'I want to learn how to play the guitar.'

4. **Acknowledge the Fear or Resistance:** Write down what's been holding you back. What is the fear or hesitation that's been stopping you from trying? This might be:
   - 'I'm afraid I'll be bad at it.'
   - 'I don't have the time or resources.'
   - 'What if I fail, and it's embarrassing?'

5. **Give Yourself Permission:** Write your permission slip. This is a personal, empowering statement granting you full permission to try without fear of judgment or failure. For example:
   - 'I give myself permission to write a novel and learn along the way.'
   - 'I give myself permission to practise, experiment and play with painting.'
   - 'I give myself permission to learn the guitar, at my own pace, and enjoy the process.'
   - Get creative with how you phrase it. The key is that it needs to be positive, punchy and potent, and it must give you permission to get it wrong, experiment, and grow.

6. **Sign and Date It:** Sign and date your permission slip. This formalises the act and makes it feel real. Make sure you put your permission slip somewhere visible. I like the fridge, toilet door, mirror, or even on your computer or phone background. This is your daily reminder to take risks and that making mistakes is a natural part of experimentation.

MISTAKES ARE OUR GREATEST LESSONS

I was invited to give a talk at a festival about my online community called the Garden Share Collective. I ran it through our food and travel blog for a few years back in 2013. It started with five people, and grew to over a couple of hundred members, all around the world. It was a monthly activity that I loved, where I got to visit gardens virtually, see what was growing, and help problem-solve any issues they were having.

The festival was one that I attended every year, so being offered a free ticket to present a talk was a no-brainer. That year I had done several talks in the area at garden expos, food festivals, and even a couple of local workshops. I was getting more confident with presenting, but this one had the largest audience, and all of my friends were going to be there.

Having no clue what to say, I tried to map out a talk as if I was writing a blog post on the topic. A 1,000-word essay was not going to cut it; I couldn't just read from a piece of paper.

Over the course of the next few months, I had to

prepare. I kept myself busy with my farm, chickens, veggies, I fell pregnant and survived the first trimester, and I worked part-time, writing and blogging while I also helped out a fellow local farmer.

Time slipped away, my online community was growing each month, and I was churning out over five blog posts a week, as well as a monthly newsletter, and helping hundreds of gardeners around the world problem-solve what was happening in their veggie patches.

There were moments where I contemplated what I was going to say, but honestly, I had all the time in the world. So obviously I left it all to the last minute. A month out from the festival, I started researching how to give a talk that didn't involve me doing a demonstration of how to grow a tomato or making the most delicious cucumber pickles. I figured they would put me in some small tent and we could all sit around and have a big ol' community discussion, my favourite way to present. It's hands-on and super interactive.

I'm not going to lie, as the time got closer, I started to freak out a little. I still didn't have a plan. And I am a girl who loves to be organised by having a plan and a list. I decided it was more important for everyone else to have the ultimate camping pack list instead, which I did share out in a cute PDF form to all my friends.

When we arrived at the festival, Roy and I took a stroll around the ground, sussing out the different tents, and where I was going to be speaking – and of course the best food places to try out. I had an empty A4 notepad and a whole day to plan my talk. I spent about ninety minutes jotting out my story, a few points on what I was supposed to talk about and, well, that was it.

I've spoken before. I knew I could wing it. But I didn't feel very confident. I had forty-five minutes to fill, and the size of the stage surprised me. The space seated over 500 people. I had spoken to a bigger crowd than that before, but not like this. What was I going to do with my hands?

Presentation day arrived. Peeling myself out of bed and unzipping our tent, I was greeted with a balmy 30°C at 7am. The temperature was forecast to reach 43°. I was pregnant, hot and bothered. I went into the festival on my own finding a cool spot to try and go over my talk again. I spent an hour procrastinating, rewriting what I already had, pretending I was going over what I was going to say. This scrappy A4 page was not helping me at all. *Fuck.*

I didn't want to do this!

I felt like a total imposter presenting at a festival that had over 100,000 people attend. Roy met up with me to walk to the stage, and he could see I was nervous. He said, 'You will be fine. You're good at this.'

I wished I believed him.

Arriving twenty minutes early to do my talk, I noticed that the guy before me was using slides. He had a lectern; he was a fucking professor! WTF. The seating area was packed, and there were people standing like sardines down the sides and at the back!

A dark cloud grew over me as I paced around in disbelief. *You've got to be kidding me, what have I got myself into? OMG OMG OMG OMG.*

PERMISSION TO GET IT WRONG

It was too late now. But I wished I had known the set-up so I could have had some visual mediums to use.

As the kind woman introduced me to the stage, I waddled up with my big belly, roasting pink face and bare feet. I was nervous as fuck. I could see a few familiar faces in the audience, but that made me even more apprehensive. I smiled and let out a little giggle. Seriously, what the fuck was I doing?

I looked at my piece of paper in the hope of regaining some sort of composure.

'Hi everyone, I'm Lizzie and I'm going to be talking about the Garden Share Collective…'

I went on to share my story of how I started gardening. I was a fourth-generation farmer at the time, and I explained how the community had grown. It took me twenty minutes of talking as fast as I could to get everything I wanted to say over and done with, so I could get off the stage. I decided to open up for questions.

A man stood up and asked, 'What is permaculture?'

I must have looked like a deer in headlights. I was not thinking straight at all. I knew what it was. But had no clue how to explain it.

'Um, it's about planting plants together to grow in harmony.' That was what I was trying to say clearly but I stumbled through a simple question.

Another question. 'What is a blog?'

OMG, who doesn't know what a blog is? This was nuts.

After the big pause with question time complete, there were still fifteen minutes left unfilled. I got off that stage as quickly as I could. A few people came over to ask more questions on the topic of gardening, which made me feel a whole lot better. I was standing with them getting my gardening on.

Being on that stage, I felt underprepared. I had just followed a man who had packed out the tent, and had slides and all. He was good! One of my friends gave me a few suggestions for next time. I brushed it off, blaming my pregnant brain for totally stuffing it up. I felt like a complete failure.

I was so happy that it was over.

What I took away from this experience, even though my ego and pride were hit hard, was that I had a lot to learn about presenting on a stage. I had never done a talk without props, let alone from behind a lectern. My talks had been interactive, on ground level, not people looking up at me.

A complete fuck-up (honestly it wasn't all bad, but at the time I was mortified). The discomfort and unease provided a great experience for me to learn. This is why our mistakes can be our greatest teachers. No matter how embarrassing or stupid I feel after a bad experience, I know for next time how to do it better.

It's in the doing.

You won't know something until you are in the moment doing the thing. Or after, like in this situation where I totally flopped, and I have never let that happen again.

LESSON DIGGING

Usually after a mega fail we beat ourselves up. I know that

has been my past reaction. I plummet to victim mode looking for things to blame, when in actual fact it was all of my own doing. This is really important to note – taking responsibility for our mistakes is an act of courage and it's completely humbling. When we own our part, we are radically accepting our path, and this opens us up for learning.

Journal Prompts

- What went wrong? List out all the bits that were a little cringy, or could have gone better.
- What would you do differently, if you could do it again?
- How can you get support or upskill for next time?
- What did you learn from your mistakes/mishaps?
- What do you need to remember for next time?
- What do you need to put in place to support you, if there is a next time?

UNCHARTED WATERS

It's pretty clear that I was underprepared for my talk. I walked off stage with fifteen minutes spare, which is an organiser's worst nightmare – dead space and an empty stage. My content was okay but I didn't have a message for the audience. I just babbled about myself and what I created. The problem was that I felt like I completely bombed and I did.

I'm going to walk you through my process to help you to dip your toes into something new and demonstrate how not to do it!

F*CK APPROVAL, YOU DON'T NEED IT!

Part One: Problem Solving

In order to solve a problem, we need to know what the problem is. Mine was that I was going to give a talk at a festival.

What I did – I got excited and looked up how to do a talk after finding out I got the gig. But then I got overwhelmed, and left it to the last minute, with many failed attempts on writing my presentation.

What I should have done – looked at it from the point of view of: fact – I am giving a talk and I have forty-five minutes on a given topic.

What is the problem I am facing (what is your unknown)?

What do I need to make it happen?

What creates anxiety is the unknown – we don't have control over the outcome, so we need to gather more information.

Part Two: Gather Resources

Next we gather resources to support us, or to provide us with the information we need. My lame attempts at researching how to give a presentation were last-minute. I had six months to prepare for my talk and I did not take it seriously (my own fault). I thought I could wing it, and that it would be enough. So I didn't invest in resources.

What I should have done is...
- Asked questions, like: what stage will I be on, and what facilities will be available to me?
- Invested in a course/mentor/teacher to help me

do a substantive talk that would last forty-five minutes (my approval seeker wanted to prove that I could do it all by myself you see).
- Seek support – someone to cheer me on outside of my circle, to give me the feedback required to improve my presentation.

Gathering resources is about getting the information we need to understand the scope of the unknown. I didn't do any of that. If you are about to dip your toes into something new, I want you to have all the relevant information you need to succeed. I don't want you to pretend, like me, that it's all fine, when in actual fact it's not.

Part Three: Evaluate

On the brink of taking that leap into the unknown, it's important to evaluate the evidence that you have gathered. To put a plan in place. Acquiring knowledge can take a bit of time – I've had to walk clients through how to get to a holiday destination solo to remove anxiety. Drawing out little pictures and lines, to show them the information they need, to do the task with confidence. It's not a bad thing, it's having the knowledge. And knowledge is wisdom.

So, once you have all the pieces in place of how to proceed and you have the facts lined up, it's now up to you.

To make a choice.

Will you proceed or will you park it? Obviously my choice was, *It's all too hard to put a talk together, I will wing it*. And I regretted my choice after. You don't need to do it as dramatically as me, but do gather your resources. Do you need to invest in them? If so, what will that take?

When you give yourself all the information, you can feel it out – remember in Chapter Three where we learned how to make informed decisions based on our gut? You can tie this in here. What emotions come up in your body when you think about taking this leap of faith? Do you want to do it? Do you have the support and facts to make it happen? Is it exciting and scary at the same time, or is it Fear Town central?

Understanding the difference between fear because we are afraid, and fear because something is dangerous, is important. History is a dark place and has a lot to answer for on this subject. It's no wonder so many of us get frightened by our own desires. The two sensations almost feel the same – *Quick, it's not safe, I need to run and hide.*

It's a cruel world, the instinct to survive is in us all.

Our mistakes are an opportunity to improve ourselves, and even change how we do things to make them work better for us. Taking responsibility for our mistakes honours what has just happened, acknowledging that there is a gap in our knowledge and that we are ready to look deeper into it. In the next chapter we are going to clear the runway for you to trust your magic and create a life beyond your wildest dreams.

Part Three
TRUST YOUR MAGIC

Chapter Eight

CLEARING THE RUNWAY TO GET WHAT YOU WANT

ONE OF THE REASONS I was so desperate to move to Scotland was its wildness and the vastness of the landscape. The endless walks that are available to be in nature. We went from having three national parks within an hour's drive from our rainforest house, with a total of twelve walks, to having 319!

But living on the west coast of the Scottish Highlands is not for the faint-hearted. The first six months I swear it rained every single day. Rain would fall delicately some days; it felt as if someone was misting your face as part of a luxury beauty regime. But on other days it would smash the windows, pounding loudly as it came in sideways, something you might see in the odd storm in Australia, but here it can go on for days – it was unlike anything I'd experienced. The number of ways moisture can fall from the sky is ridiculous, from hail to snow to sleet. For someone who used to record how much rain they had each month, seeing it every day was a whole new experience.

Investing in waterproofs for school pickup was essential; each afternoon all the parents wait in whatever the weather throws at them. They were hardy. Yes, they would complain about the rain, snow or hailstones. This was my new normal; in Australia we used to hide from this kind of weather and wait for it to pass. Here, they just got on with it, like it was nothing. It was normal.

One of the rules I have always lived by is that one should lead by example. Opening up my Cognitive Behavioural Therapy practice, I got a fast introduction to Scottish culture, its problems and outdoor tips. These people are stoic sometimes to their detriment, but they can put on a jacket and get out in any weather, and just do the thing.

Each week I would take Monday and Wednesday mornings off for a walk. I needed this space to think, to ground myself, but also to calm my nervous system. Every month, as I got busier and busier with clients, the weather always tested my commitment to self.

Weather shouldn't be an excuse. The first saying I learned here was that there is no such thing as bad weather, just the wrong clothing. It still makes me smile, and it is so true. If it's raining, and you want to go out, get dressed for it. If it's cold, get dressed for it. Makes sense.

Stop waiting.

It wasn't long before I decided to restart my Couch to 5k journey – a running app that I had dabbled with in Australia, where I never made it past week four, because they made me run for five-minute blocks. Back then I used to run in the morning around 9am and the heat was a killer. The thick air on the flats was humid and it sucked the life out of me every time. No wonder I hated running. I hadn't run since I was in high school and taking it up at the age of thirty-seven made me question my sanity. Plus, I can give you all the excuses about why my body hated running – wiggly bits, bras to control the boob sway, and the sweat. Yuk!

The reason why I wanted to start running in Scotland was to help me improve my uphill adventures. Our luxurious paths in Australia, which meander through forests, mountains and hills, are not quite as steep as those in Scotland. Here, they are devil's staircases. There is one track that I walk called 'the heart attack track' because of its sheer verticality. It's a killer, but it seems that most tracks involve going up; they are often stony paths and require at least fifty breaks to get to the top.

Yes, a slight exaggeration, but it feels like that, needing to stop every five minutes because you're so puffed. I wanted to keep up with my youngest, who can scale a mountain in no time, no sweat and with complete ease. He had to constantly wait for Mummy to catch up, and then sit while my lungs felt like they could breathe again. I didn't want that anymore.

Determined to make this life change towards getting healthier, my goal was to make it past week five on the Couch to 5K app. I wanted to improve my endurance, and be able to go longer, without as many breaks up those hills. It started off relatively easy, one-minute jogs, then to two minutes. I paced them well and each week the times would increase.

The weather would often encroach on my plans, and put them back a day or two, but I was still out there doing it. The day before the dreaded five-minute run, I had a client come in who was talking about cycling home again after work. I, being super curious, asked all the practical questions around it, because I was like – *What happens when it's raining?* His reply is something I've never forgotten.

'Commit to getting wet.'

Yes, you can imagine my facial expression here, confused, slightly screwed up, questioning if this guy had lost his mind. He was raised here – he had inside knowledge that I didn't have.

If you are going to go out in Scotland, there is a good chance you might get soaked, so if it happens, do it well. I loved this. The reason I love this so much is that it takes commitment and I think that is a solid reminder for all of us: that in order to create change we must commit to our practice.

Self-discipline sounds super boring, and some days it is. I set out to establish a 6am morning writing practice, because I wanted to get better at writing. I had a project in mind that I wanted to work on, but it wasn't easy.

When I was eighteen, I was in the thick of art school and was still creating all kinds of weird and wonderful things. I used to screen-print my own clothes and one of the shirts said, 'I'm not a morning person'.

It's still true today. Even though I've had jobs that start at 6am in the past, my body has always disliked being woken up abruptly. The sun on my face is always welcome to stir me, but an alarm making all the noises sucks. Yes, it's called life and it's not an excuse. But it kept me up at night worried I was going to sleep through my alarm, which inevitably made it harder to get up in the morning. Even after committing to my practice for three months, I still held a grudge even as my body clock slowly started to sync to this new pattern.

There are no interruptions at that time of the morning, no kids up yet who need feeding. Just me, a light, a notebook and pen. My alarm would sound and I would immediately get up, not leaving any time for my head to kick in and tell me how cosy my bed was. Because my bed is really cosy, super comfortable and warm! And the outside world is cold and requires me to put on additional clothes that are far from body temperature in the hope of keeping myself warm.

The fight was always real when the alarm went off – should I stay or should I get out of bed? That one thought, that one decision, can change everything. That is why it takes commitment and self-discipline to get what you want. My writing project of writing for just one hour a day saw my word count go from zero to 10,000 in a matter of months. I completed what I set out to do. Yes, it was challenging; yes, there were obstacles to overcome – but the sense of achievement was worth it.

In this chapter we are going to talk about procrastination, overcoming obstacles, and getting our mindset on board to create the life we want. This is the beginning of self-trust, to back yourself and your dreams.

F*CK APPROVAL, YOU DON'T NEED IT!

What self-commitment looks like

I'm a list writer; there is a small piece of me that still carries anxiety about not being prepared for a situation. It's funny because I also married a list writer. We both love a list. Anything from the ultimate camping packing list to what we hope to achieve for the year is list-worthy. Roy has always challenged me and inspired me. And after we went travelling to Japan in 2019 he realised that he wished he had learned more of the language. There could have been so many culinary delights available if only we had known how to read menus near the markets. With our next trip being planned to China, he worked out a way to learn Chinese that worked for him. But it wasn't long before he realised that there was not enough time in the day. He left for work early before the kids got up, which gifted him early finishes. He wanted to give them his time and attention. They too would check the time for when Dad was going to arrive home, knowing that the fun would begin. By the time he went to bed, he was exhausted and couldn't concentrate on his handmade flash cards. He decided to get up earlier to study before work.

At first I honestly didn't think he would stick it out.

I assumed this from my own personal experience of not being an early riser. Supporting him, we made sure he had everything he needed to make this practice work. Five years on, Roy still gets up super early and practises his language.

That is self-commitment, and we can all learn from him.

ACKNOWLEDGE PROCRASTINATION

Perfectionism is procrastination's best friend. Double that with a list of excuses and no one is getting anywhere fast. The reason why many of us are endlessly running around is that we get distracted. Procrasta-cleaning is real. I can't start writing unless the house is clean. I can't start running because I need new shoes. There is always something in the way.

My biggest weaknesses used to be procrasta-cleaning and procrasta-organising. When I decided to write a book, it took a lot for me to get on board with the project. I was excited about doing it, but my commitment levels were far from gold medal worthy.

Apparently, I needed to have a clear kitchen and a clean living room before I could work. The clothes need to be sorted or washed. I would spend an hour or so making sure the space was ready every day so I could get my laptop out and start typing. For any creative person, the curse of a blank page still remains. Which would then have me working out what I needed to do, writing the list, and then breaking down the list, all in order to get me in the zone. Usually, by this time it was lunchtime, which meant I needed a break – another healthy distraction, another ploy against me.

Arriving back at my laptop, I would then doom-scroll on social media and check my email for the eighteenth time. Time slipped away, and what was left was spent on a single paragraph, reworking it until it was right, over and over, before I had to race out of the door to get my kids.

Procrastination is a distraction.

Which for me always leads to frustration about not doing the thing I wanted to do, and not getting as much done as I had hoped. What I did have was a functional house that was clean and tidy. That cycle of following an 'old rule' because I believed that it was important. I forgot to update it to match what I was currently doing.

I remember reading a book about our energy levels, and how it's important to use it in the best way possible. If you are a morning person who gets up and wants to hit the road running, you should use that energy for the things you want. Why burn it all out on stupid shit that doesn't bring you a sense of fulfilment?

For example, Roy realised that his brain worked better in the morning and could absorb information then, so it was the best time for him to learn language based on his energy.

This concept of using your energy wisely was everything. I too am a morning person, but only after a cup of tea – then it's go-time! My energy dips around 2pm as my brain begins to slow down. So why waste my most productive time on cleaning the house when I could be writing?

I call this concept Prime Time. It's where we use our energy for good. It was a simple flip to swap my house duties with writing. It took time for me to relax about the toys on the floor, but it worked. I somehow would smash out way more words in the morning than I would in the afternoons when my brain had stopped working.

The trick with Prime Time is to allocate yourself a few hours to the task at hand, where your energy is aligned to the task, and then to focus on it without distraction. I've installed blockers on my laptop for social media and email during my Prime Time, so that I will stay on task.

Self-discipline is again our greatest ally.

Watching the Olympics always blows my mind. There are people in this world who have abilities far beyond what we know. They have a sense of determination, grit, and self-discipline to make dreams a reality. We have a lot to learn from them.

Much can be said about the athletes that compete. What we see in a five-minute or ten-second performance is the end result of years and years of dedication, training and mastery. Practice is everything, perfection is what they aim and aspire to, but they know that, just like us, we are all human and we can only give our best on the day with what we have got.

My running practice has opened up my lungs and gets me up the Scottish mountains with more ease. I'm still stopping to catch my breath, but not as much as before. It's improving slowly. When we decide what we want we can focus our energy on it, and that helps us to allocate our Prime Time towards making it happen.

OVERCOMING OBSTACLES EXERCISE

Here is where we need to get real about all the things that are getting in the way of our dreams.

Overcoming obstacles helps to build our resilience, strengthens our determination, and promotes a positive mindset. By addressing the things that get in the way, we become aware of tweaks that we need to make. Think of this as clearing the runway for success.

F*CK APPROVAL, YOU DON'T NEED IT!

I'm going to talk through my 6am morning writing practice from the time when I was 'not a morning person', to now, when I am organised and committed to my practice. So that split-second decision between staying in bed or not is no longer an issue.

The first morning I dragged my feet as I came down the stairs. It was quarter past six before I even sat down with my notebook and pen. But I was impressed that I had actually got up. Not a perfect start, since I spent most of my time faffing about. I started off being concerned about actually getting up instead of writing. What I learned (see, our experiences are our greatest teachers) was that I needed to be more prepared. That same evening, I made sure that my notebook and pen were on the table, ready for me to pick up as soon as I made it to the couch. I also decided to make sure I had extra layers to wear within arm's reach, for as soon as I got up.

As the week went on, my husband kept trying to engage in conversation with me at this ungodly hour. Yes, he simply wanted a 'Good morning' back. But I was so unimpressed about being up anyway – he wasn't meant to be talking at me at 6am in the morning. While he sat there with his flash cards, having already been up for an hour prior to my arrival, I would pretend he wasn't there so I could just go into my writing zone.

That was what I was there to do! He knew that – why was it such a big deal for me to crack a smile before 7am? Writing, not hanging out! This led to me having a conversation about my needs. It felt so silly and selfish. I was demanding he ignore me, and let me flop on the

CLEARING THE RUNWAY TO GET WHAT YOU WANT

couch to write without interruption between the strict hours I was meant to be writing. Oh boundaries, we love you, but sometimes you test the best of us.

Obstacles are all the things that make us second-guess our choices in the moment. We want our choice to be easy. So we need to set ourselves up for it. Establishing this new practice, I noticed what had to change from the very first day; there were a few other hurdles that came along too. But I was showing up for it, I was committing myself to the practice, and through my observations, I could make changes to make it easier for myself.

Overcoming our obstacles is in the doing; it's clearing the runway for success.

There was a ten-month period where I worked in a cafe, which required me to start at 6am. I would cycle to work five days a week. I knew exactly how long it took me to ride, which I then worked back from, to the time my alarm would go off – making it easy for this non-morning person to arrive. I ensured I had enough time to get dressed, brush my teeth, do my hair, and go to the toilet before putting my helmet on. It became an easy autopilot routine that served me well.

Here is what I want you to do. If you have been putting off doing something, I want you to write down all the reasons why, and then face those excuses head on. Give yourself a loving, stern talking-to, and get your mindset back on board, and let's make a plan.

I want you to write down a timeline to make the task a reality. Here is an example of my 6am morning writing practice.

Night before:	Notebook and pen ready on table, slippers at the bottom of the stairs, big cup next to sink, big woolly jumper and trackie bottoms next to bed.
5.50am:	Alarm goes off.
5.51am:	Get layers on, walk downstairs, get my slippers on, go to the toilet, go to the kitchen, get a drink of water and make my way to the couch to make a nest with blankets.
6am:	Pick up my notebook and pen. Write, write and write.
7am:	Mum mode – feed kids and get ready for school/day.
8.30am:	School run.

I worked through every obstacle that might have stopped me. Hubby was up before me, so he would turn the heater on so the room where I wrote wasn't Baltic. The little things matter.

Journal Prompts:

- *What are the obstacles getting in your way that are stopping/delaying you from your task?*
- *What do you need to do to clear the runway to make doing the task easier?*
- *Write down your timeline to achieve the task.*

MINDSET, MINDSET, MINDSET

Having a positive mindset requires us to manage our negative thoughts, by understanding what triggers them.

CLEARING THE RUNWAY TO GET WHAT YOU WANT

This is why boundaries are powerful for protecting our energy, and we will go over that in the next chapter. But first we need to talk about the weight of our words. And taking baby steps towards change.

I had just been dumped by my first big love. We worked at the same restaurant, and my shift was finally coming to an end. Pretending that my feelings were not hurt, I went deep into a conversation with the new girl. To be honest, she wasn't a girl, she was a woman, and her charismatic personality intrigued me. She asked us all if we knew anyone who wanted to trade some time to help her in her garden, for a Japanese Nine Star Ki reading. Having always been super interested in astrology and anything a little alternative, I instantly said yes.

The following week I spent the whole day in her garden weeding, a task I enjoyed. A few days later I was invited for tea on her verandah. The house was amazing – her decor was swoon-worthy, from antiques to plants, and the house smelt delicious with essential oil in the air. She was living my dream, and now I was going to have my astrology read, Japanese-style.

What was a beautiful exchange led to a great friendship. The weeding went on for a few weeks, while our conversations over tea grew longer and longer, and I learned so much. One day I was rattling off how I was doubting myself about where my life was going. I felt low. Instantly, the garden lady pulled me up on my words.

She explained that it matters how we speak to others about ourselves. I felt confused. I had this drive within me that worked a little like this: I did something >> I found what was wrong with it >> then I would try to fix it or make it better.

I was constantly looking for faults; I was never enough; even my inner dialogue was wired that way.

To be caught saying mean things about myself was a little confronting. But it was done with so much care and consideration. I saw it as a lesson and we talked about magnets. How positive words attract good into your life and also how our words affect our vibration. Yes, it was the garden lady who introduced me to Dr Emoto and his mind-blowing water experiment. We agreed that I would no longer speak badly of myself and that if it happened again she would pull me up on it.

It took a while to practise not bad-mouthing myself or playing down my skills. As a twenty-two-year-old, it seemed so normal. Everyone around me body-shamed themselves for hours before going out for a drink. We all questioned our power as women, and the roles we should be following.

Normalising negative talk and thinking occurs when the people around us do the same. The garden lady invited me to change this, instead of mirroring that language. What I realised over the coming weeks, when I stopped feeding my inner bitch with endless negativity, was how many other people allowed the negative thoughts to tear them apart.

Mindset is everything; when we are positive and open ourselves up to failures from a place of compassion, we can do anything. But when we see ourselves through a negative lens, it's disaster town.

Cultivating a positive mindset requires us to see the good in things. It's retraining the brain.

STOP NEGATIVE SELF-TALK

Life is too short to waste energy on negative self-talk.

From the way we speak, to the way we play down who we are, managing our negative thoughts requires us to monitor our emotional reactions. When clients come to me explaining that they want to be happier, they often can't describe what happiness actually looks like for them. All they know is that how they feel right now is not how they want to be living their lives.

Here is what comes out of their mouths next...

- *I'm overly emotional, and I need to stop.*
- *I don't want to bother anyone with my stuff.*
- *I want to be normal, like everyone else.*

It can be hard to notice how these statements are actually the result of negative thinking. They sound more like facts. We live by them. Rules, right?

If we go back to Chapter Two and apply our fact-checking process, then we can see that these statements are not true. But we keep saying them to ourselves.

Managing negativity requires us to look at what triggers that spiral of thought. We live in a world that is very noisy, screens everywhere, information everywhere, everything is instant. Our environment has a dramatic impact on us. What we consume influences our thoughts.

Growing up without social media or the internet was a blessing, one that I'm very grateful for. I've always used the online space for one thing, and that is business. Social media was originally designed to connect people, right? Friends were able to stay in touch, families who live long-distance could easily keep up to date, and we all became accessible.

However, it soon turned into a product that could be sold, and it became a multimillion-dollar industry, very different from how we originally used it.

It used to be a place to invite our mates round for a party, and post the aftermath photos.

Then it became a place to shop, get the news, and the latest gossip.

Scrolling became far too easy.

When my days of partying hard were officially over, I was a mother. I fell into the trap of wasting time scrolling through all the mummy bloggers I followed online.

They made mum life look so whimsical and easy. Their cute toddlers posed in the kitchen with a splodge of yoghurt delicately placed on their cheek as if they had just made a mess but in their Sunday finest. The top line of the post would go something like this: *How to get your kid to eat vegetables!* OMG, I used to take Isla's wooden highchair outside onto the veranda and, if the weather allowed it, she sat in the nude. I would give her a bowl of yoghurt which, within ten minutes, was all over her face, through her hair, and flicked all over the ground, me and the shed walls. I took a photo once of her with a spoon in hand, proud as punch and yogurt everywhere. There was no filter or glamorous outfit in sight. But to this day I can look at that photo and relive a memory of how we used to roll when she was little.

It made me wonder how these Insta mums did it. Cue self-doubt, and a negativity spiral approaching.

CLEARING THE RUNWAY TO GET WHAT YOU WANT

Their kids only ate organic food, they were somehow size eight again after having a baby, doing yoga in their picturesque houses while their cute-as-a-button bub was on the floor, with its lovey-dovey eyes looking back at her in her organic yoga wear. This was enough to sink me into a rabbit hole of negative thinking.

Why doesn't my life look like that?

Why don't my kids sit still long enough to get their picture taken without trashing what they are wearing?

What am I doing wrong?

Why don't I fit into my yoga leggings yet?

My social feed became my nemesis.

My reality looked like me in the veggie patch covered in mud, chasing our chooks with a mum bun and a T-shirt that had at least six different spills or stains on it from the day.

I needed it to stop.

I started placing boundaries around how I used my phone – we will talk about them in the next chapter. That worked for a bit, as I limited my use; however, it was what I was seeing that was the issue.

I remember someone reminding me that you should face your triggers. I agreed. Absolutely. However, why do we need to live each day in a headspace of negative mind talk when we can do something about it? The guilt from unfollowing over a hundred accounts ripped through me. *Would they know that I did it? Would they think I disliked them?* It wasn't personal; it was for my mental well-being.

Was I avoiding conflict by not facing my triggers? Was I simply meant to persevere each time I opened up my app? It's common for people-pleasers to dislike the thought of upsetting the status quo, and I didn't want it to affect anyone by my actions. The burden!

I did it anyway.

Days later, checking my messages felt less stressful. I was no longer protecting myself with a heavy-duty forcefield that was weighing me down to make sure my mind didn't spiral out of control. My behaviours changed. I deleted the apps from my phone, and only used them during business hours to check messages, and interact with the people who inspired me. I began to cultivate a healthy use of social media, which made me value the importance of relationships, both the ones we have in person, but also my relationship with myself.

I stopped looking at others to set my standard of living.

I stopped following people who made me feel 'less than'.

I stopped consuming content that made me doubt who I was.

Managing negativity is about being discerning as to what you let into your life. It's learning to recognise your triggers, and then doing something about it. It's exploring solutions to help stop negative thinking taking over.

- Replace late-night binge-watching of Netflix with going to bed early
- Replace influencers with inspiring creators.
- Replace toxic friends with mentors.
- Replace complaining with gratitude.
- Replace overthinking with taking action.
- Replace sad songs with ones that make you want to dance.

CLEARING THE RUNWAY TO GET WHAT YOU WANT

- *Replace negative people with people that reflect back how you want to feel and be.*
- *Replace keeping busy with being intentional.*

I want to remind you that negative thoughts are not 'bad'. They are just thoughts that take you to a place you don't want to be. Explore that. Don't punish yourself for it happening, but question the trigger. What's behind your discomfort? Is there something you can do about it? Does it need time? Does it need healing? Does it need a boundary?

ACTION PLAN

Here is where the fun begins. Learning to trust your crazy. When I started a 6am writing practice, I didn't know how it was going to turn out. When I decided to start running to improve my fitness, I had no clue how long it was going to take to see results. When I decided to move my family from sunny Australia to Scotland, I didn't know if it was the smartest thing to do.

All I knew was that I wanted it, and I wanted it so bad, I would do anything for it.

Like any good plan, we need a final destination, and to know where we are currently at. This way we can work out how to get from A to B. I'm going to walk you through our crazy move to the other side of the world.

THE START: What's happening in your life and what do you deeply desire? For us it was that we were seeking something new, something that felt expansive, and we wanted a change from the life we had.

THE DESTINATION: Snow-capped peaks, lounge-room view.

THE PLAN: Find a job, work out how we were going to move. I wrote down a three-stage plan which I hung on the wall to give me a daily reminder.

OBSTACLES: Visas, border passes, car hire, downsizing a family of four, shipping, schools, bank accounts, somewhere to live on arrival and buying a car.

Call me organised, or someone who considers every possibility. There is a side of me that loves to test my limits, where the rule book goes out the window. Logic is pushed to the side, as I do whatever it takes, outlining all the details. Yet, Roy likes to remind me when I go overboard with a plan, to stay open and flexible. And that it's okay to not have it all worked out, that we just need the essentials to get the ball rolling.

Clear the runway.
Don't control the journey.
Be flexible, follow the path.
Fine-tune.
We are all here working it out as we go.

CLEARING THE RUNWAY TO GET WHAT YOU WANT

CREATE YOUR ACTION PLAN

Grab yourself a piece of paper or journal and work through the following questions:

1. Discovering What You Truly Want

- **What does my ideal life look like in three years?** Describe a day in your life as vividly as possible, three years from now.
- **What areas of my life currently feel 'meh' or unfulfilling?** Identify specific areas (relationships, career, health, etc.) and what's missing or not working within them.
- **When do I feel the most alive, inspired, or passionate?** Reflect on moments when you truly felt your authentic self.
- **If I had no limitations (money, time, fear), what would I pursue?** Let yourself dream big without holding back.
- **What do I value most in life?** List core values that matter to you, and consider how they align with your current life.

2. Defining Your Personal Goals

- **What can I do to bridge the gap between my current reality and my dream life?** Be specific about goals that address areas you want to improve.
- **What does success mean to me?** Describe success in your terms, not society's expectations.
- **What goals make me feel excited and scared at**

the same time?** Often, these are the ones worth pursuing!

3. *Creating a Plan of Action*

- **What does a 'magical' life mean to me?** Define what a life full of joy, purpose, and passion looks like to you.
- **What are the biggest challenges or obstacles to reaching my goals?** Consider both external and internal roadblocks.

4. *Mapping Out Steps for Transformation*

- **What small action can I take this week that moves me closer to my goals?** Focus on tiny, manageable steps that build momentum.
- **What daily practices or rituals can I implement to stay connected to my vision?** Think about journaling, meditation, or daily affirmations.
- **Who can support or guide me on this journey?** Consider mentors, friends, or communities that align with your aspirations.
- **What do I need to learn or improve to bring my dreams closer to reality?** Identify any skills, knowledge, or personal growth areas to work on.
- **How can I celebrate small wins along the way?** Plan ways to reward yourself for progress, no matter how small.

5. *Committing to Long-Term Change*

- **What kind of person do I need to become to

live this magical life? Reflect on how you'll need to grow and evolve personally. Think about your essence or Big Deal Energy.
- **How can I ensure that I remain focused on my goals during challenging times?** Think about strategies to stay motivated when things get tough. Identify your non-negotiables to keep you on track.
- **What does self-compassion look like for me when I stumble?** Create a plan to be kind to yourself when things don't go perfectly.

Creating new practices and chasing after your dreams requires self-trust that things will work out. Self-discipline and commitment will see slow but positive change while impatience is a symptom of expectations. Life is for living, and for experiences that bring us joy. Now it's time to set some boundaries to keep those promises to yourself.

Chapter Nine
EMPOWERMENT THROUGH BOUNDARIES & PROTECTION

WHENEVER A FRIEND IS IN my neighbourhood, I always like to make the effort to cross paths with them, because who knows when that might happen again? At this point in my life, it's hectic and busy with two small kids in tow. Each day can feel like a year.

I was sitting in the sun at a funky pavement café with a dear friend. It was a sacred moment, where the outside noise of the city didn't distract me from our conversation. Loving every moment of adult conversation, I was thrilled when she spontaneously invited me to the event she was speaking at. Having a friendly face in the audience always puts me at ease too. Plus, she asked if I could double as a photographer, as she knew I was pretty handy with a camera. A total no-brainer for me – a free event, a night off from mum duties, and another opportunity to hang with my friend.

EMPOWERMENT THROUGH BOUNDARIES & PROTECTION

I didn't even have to think about it. I would do anything for them. I responded instantly with 'Of course, I would love to.'

Arriving at the venue early as arranged, I scanned the room and noticed that it wasn't ready to welcome fifty people. The organiser looked flustered, while the additional helper was rushing around the room arranging furniture. My inner organiser, whom you met in Chapter Three, set to work. A ninja skill that had seen me run several events in the past couldn't unsee the list of what needed to be done.

Within a second, I couldn't help myself, and I jumped in ready to save the day.

It wasn't my job, but I was happy to take on the responsibility, because I didn't want my mate's event to flop. Moving quickly around the room, I rearranged plants on the stage, to make it look more visually appealing, and organised flowers that were just left on a bench, with no vase in sight. I fussed over the food, to make it look bigger and better. What happened in that half an hour was that I buried myself knee-deep in the work. I completely depleted my energy, and I was knackered by the time people began to arrive. No one had asked me to do any of that. I took it upon myself – a selfless act of love, right? Or was I seeking approval for my efforts?

I couldn't rest until the event finished. I was on duty, with my eyes wide open to monitor everything in the room. Yes, I take things very seriously. It's my Aussie country gal work ethic. We're designed like workhorses to see the job through to the end and put 120 per cent in at all times.

Afterwards, everyone looked to me to help coordinate the pack-down! It wasn't until about an hour later I realised that, while I was exhausted, the people around me looked glamorous as fuck.

How did this happen?

How did I let this happen?

Sipping on a cocktail in the bar around the corner with a few people from the event, trying to make small talk with yet another new person felt like the hardest thing ever.

Why did I always make it my responsibility to help others, to my own detriment? I thought back to the time I went to work at 6am in the morning after someone called in sick and my boss needed me. I had the world's worst hangover because it was meant to be my day off, but what was my response?

'Of course.' I rolled out of bed and went to work.

Or the time when I was having coffee with a friend, and her daughter ran away from our table over to the other side of the café – my immediate response was to go and chase after her, allowing her plenty of space to explore safely. And do you know what that friend said to me?

'This is why I'm so fucking lucky. I have people like you in my life who do stuff for me. It's awesome.'

What the actual fuck?

I give and I give. I do it because I see it as kindness, as an act of service, as respect. (Yes, my love language is acts of service. How did you guess?)

Flopping into bed that night, a sigh slipped out, as I realised the physical and energetic toll of my actions. I was absolutely knackered. I had walked away from a free round of cocktails because I felt drained from taking on all that extra responsibility.

So why did I do it?

I didn't want my friend to be let down, so my sense of duty kicked in, which then triggered a whole lot of guilt about being invited to attend free of charge. So I made up for that by taking on responsibility as a way to prove that I deserved the ticket.

Boo, my approval addiction won.

I burned myself out for someone else. And you know what, I never even got a thank you.

That kept me awake!

And it's all because I didn't have any fucking boundaries.

I didn't see the value in protecting myself or my energy because I could only see others' needs. Also, it was totally my own fault, and we are going to explore this as we go deep on boundaries.

A boundary is something we put in place to exercise our right to protect ourselves, acknowledging our values and limitations.

This experience demonstrated to me how quickly my energy could get sucked away, which led to rather unpleasant emotions. I felt like shit, and that sucked, so the next day I was wiped out. It didn't help that my mind was rerunning through the events of the night before.

WHAT IS A HEALTHY BOUNDARY?

The word 'boundary' serves as an indicator for our limits of anything, whether material or emotional, signifying something we don't tolerate. A boundary is where you draw a line of what is and what is not important to you. It clearly states your values and limitations.

Boundaries can be set in many areas of our life including: our energy, time, financial, emotional, mental or physical.

I like to think of boundaries as little white picket fences surrounding your space, with gates that you can open or close whenever you need to let energy flow in or out. Those are completely controlled by you.

When you close the gate, you stop the flow of anything coming in that you don't want. When the gate is closed, you also protect yourself from having all your energy sucked out of you. We will talk about energy vampires later in this chapter.

When you unconsciously leave the gate open, you are exposing your lack of personal standards. Which makes it really easy to take advantage of you, because you are so willing to compromise yourself for others. And we don't want that for you anymore.

When we set boundaries, we are telling the world that we understand our personal needs, and how we want to be treated. Boundaries are a beautiful reminder that we are all equals, and that we don't need to play small for others.

There are two distinct kinds of boundaries:

INTERNAL BOUNDARIES

These are the boundaries we set for ourselves, by us, for us. Think of them as your non-negotiables. The rules you live by to protect your time, energy and headspace. They don't need to be shared with another. They are the promises you make to yourself.

They can look like:
- *I don't use my phone until I get to work in the mornings*
- *I don't take phone calls after 8pm*
- *I don't go out when I'm tired and desperately need rest*
- *I won't engage in conversations about body weight*
- *I will move my body daily*
- *I won't talk about politics or money with my parents*

When internal boundaries need to be set:
- *When the source of your frustration or resentment is caused by your own actions of over-giving, over-committing or sacrificing yourself.*
- *When you take on other people's emotional baggage and energy and find it overwhelming*
- *When external boundaries are not working but you still need to ensure that your needs are being met (this can look like creating distance away from the cause)*

The truth is, we can save ourselves an incredible amount of time, energy, and difficult conversations by getting better at honouring our own internal boundaries first.

Imagine if I had had the audacity to not help unless asked. What kind of boundary is that? Well, it's one that

I now live by, thanks to this event. It's not my place to rescue others unless they ask me too. Obviously, if it was life and death, I would totally jump in without waiting for an invitation.

I want you to see that internal boundaries are little promises that pack a lot of power. They demonstrate how much we value ourselves, and what we are willing to do to maintain our own emotional well-being. Seeing these boundaries comes with practice, like all things. But when mastered, these power bombs are what define us – they can make us strong, confident, and completely unstoppable.

They are new rules for you to live by – ones designed for you, and by you!

For example:

- *I will not be the middle person between two people – friends or family members*
- *I will not invest in friendships that suck away my energy*
- *I don't over-commit to social activities because I value my family time*

EXTERNAL BOUNDARIES

These are the boundaries that require us to communicate and speak with others. This is where big conversations happen, demonstrating how we wish to be treated, explaining how we value ourselves, all to teach the other person/s about your boundaries.

They can look like:

- *I don't like it when you talk about body image and your weight, as I find it triggering*

EMPOWERMENT THROUGH BOUNDARIES & PROTECTION

- Saying no to an extra shift on Friday because you have other plans
- Sharing that you don't like to be hugged or touched in a particular way
- That you can't make it to a party because you have a date with yourself
- That you don't tolerate people who are not open to equality
- Speaking up when you see something that you don't agree with

When external boundaries need to be set:
- When your limits are being crossed by another person. You'll know when, hands down! Usually, big feelings and emotions come up; they stir an awareness within you that you have been wronged, and that this is not how you want to feel

External boundaries require a lot from us, in that we need to speak up for ourselves, to communicate our limitations, and to educate the other person on our personal standards. This means that, through telling them, they now have this information, and can adjust accordingly. Talking is key and we have a whole chapter on that next.

In the previous story, even if someone had asked me to help set up, I could have said no, but obviously that wasn't the case at all. Setting a boundary with someone can be as easy as saying no, and we will talk about that soon. First, let's look at how to set a boundary.

F*CK APPROVAL, YOU DON'T NEED IT!

HOW TO SET AND MAINTAIN BOUNDARIES

As individuals, we do not have a duty to look after everyone we know. We don't need to be the one to rush to the emergency, save the day, or prioritise the importance of others over ourselves all the time.

Boundaries are the greatest gift we can give ourselves.

Yes, I know it can seem somewhat scary to finally draw the line in the sand and to stand our ground. But it is for our greater good and enables us to do life better. Yes, we might be met with resistance at first, but that is what happens when we come across people who ignore or don't accept boundaries. Just remember that we have also been there. It evokes feelings of abandonment or selfishness, which makes us question ourselves. Boundaries bring up a lot of triggers, especially when we make them and stand by them.

Setting boundaries is a way for us to gain more personal space, time, energy, and things we want. We can place boundaries in all areas of our life. They improve our confidence, give us greater self-esteem, a nicer living environment, and more independence.

Creating effective boundaries will come with practice, patience, and a lot of trial and error to fine-tune them. Boundaries have enabled me to live a life where I feel free, surrounded by people who support me and the work I do. They allow me to say a firm no, without feeling guilty.

Step 1: Understand Your Limits

Before setting your boundaries, you need to be clear about your values, and recognise what you find unacceptable.

EMPOWERMENT THROUGH BOUNDARIES & PROTECTION

These are the things you won't tolerate, knowing your limits. For example, I won't tolerate someone talking over the top of me, or anyone else. My limit is the moment when someone has rudely interrupted or hijacked the conversation. That is when a boundary would need to be set.

Our boundaries are the hard lines we draw, but there are lots of things we still might tolerate that might get under our skin. It's important for you to know your own limitations because no one can tell you how you feel about something.

The Key Players – Values, Limits & Tolerances

Write down a list of values – the rules you want to live your life by. Here are a few examples:

- **RESPONSIBILITY** – Be accountable for your actions and commitments.
- **INTEGRITY** – Act with honesty and strong moral principles.
- **RESPECT** – Treat others with kindness, consideration, and understanding.
- **OPENNESS** – Be open to new ideas, perspectives, and experiences.
- **GENEROSITY** – Share your resources, time, and care with others.

Write down a list of limitations (these are your hard 'No's!). Here are a few examples:

- Being touched inappropriately.
- Being spoken to disrespectfully or like a child.

- Engaging in or witnessing gossip and malicious talk.
- Being used or taken advantage of.
- Body shaming in any form.
- Racism, sexism, or any form of discrimination.
- Excessive work demands that infringe on personal time.

Write down a list of what you are willing to tolerate
- Occasional lateness from close friends or family.
- Constructive criticism, when given respectfully.
- Differences in opinion, provided there's mutual respect.
- Minor, unintentional mistakes, as long as accountability is taken.
- Emotional outbursts, if they're not abusive and are followed by apologies.

Can you see how boundaries serve to protect us? This is important. Let's explore this a little deeper, by looking at these questions:
- What situations or behaviours make me feel uncomfortable or stressed?
- What physical and emotional signs indicate that you have reached your limit?

Step 2: Identify The Boundary You Need To Place

Most likely you can already identify a situation that you need to change. If you are anything like me, it's been rubbing you up the wrong way for a while, and you have a gut feeling about it. Not all situations are so easy to read and this is where we need to practise awareness. Just like when I realised that I was saying yes to my boss all the time so as not to disappoint her. Being aware of this was a skill that I developed over time. I learned to pause for a moment before reacting, doing or talking.

A great way to check in is to ask yourself, 'Am I okay with this?'

When dealing with boundaries in real time it's important to look for a rise in emotion – frustration, resentment, anger, etc. These feelings can help us to notice quickly that a boundary is required.

Next, we need to ask ourselves, is this a boundary we need to set with someone else or with ourselves?

Is it an external or an internal boundary?

IF IT'S EXTERNAL: who are you setting the boundary with? What do you need to say to educate the other person of your boundary?

IF IT'S INTERNAL: What practice/rule do you need to implement to set the boundary (i.e. not using your phone before bed, etc.).

THE KEY QUESTION: What can you do right now to assert your choice or needs? (This is an action.) Clue – this is often something that you know you need to do, but that you have been putting off. This step is about opening our eyes to how we are responding to those around us, and honouring what we need to do for us.

Step 3: Communicate Your Boundary

This is the part most of us get nervous about. It requires us to talk about our needs, giving voice to our desires and standards. When we share them with others, we are educating them. As soon as we do this, we put down the weight that we carry on our shoulders. Unspoken boundaries are what often cause us stress, and that stress is often the reason we snap, out of frustration.

It takes courage to acknowledge that we are not okay with something.

And it takes even greater courage to communicate that boundary.

All right, now to the tricky bit. You have said no, defended yourself, stated your terms, and asked assertively. Now, take a big breath because this is the moment we totally deserve a little kudos. It is where we stand our ground in the emptiness of space and time, and wait for the response from the other person, or people. Scary as fuck, I know, but don't feel like you need to fill the gap with words. I can't stress how important it is to wait for the response. It can sometimes feel like a minute has passed, when in reality it was two seconds. The wait is worth it and you might be surprised at the outcome.

Step 4: Evaluate The Response Received

Not everyone is going to respond the way you want them to, when you say what you need to say, without excuses or justifying yourself. So, we need to take a moment to digest the response once we have received it.

If all goes well, you will get a green light and work out all the details to move forward.

But if you hit a red light, and are met with negativity and push-back, you will need to consider what you do next. This might look like compromising, asserting our boundary again, providing another solution or giving them more information, to help them see our perspective.

This step is a brilliant exercise in learning to deal with conflict (I know, it's uncomfortable and most likely your worst nightmare), which also strengthens our communication skills. It provides a space to practise reflecting back what the other person has said, and discussing the situation openly.

Just a final note on creating boundaries: start small. If saying no is hard, then practise. Perhaps set some boundaries with your partner and kids, like being able to go to the toilet in peace, without interruptions. Tackle the small things; voice what it is you need or want, and focus on how it can support you.

POWER OF SAYING NO

When Kelly moved in, I was beyond excited to have a fellow woman in our shared house, to break up the dynamic of boozy nights and parties with the three boys I had come to know and love. I had failed at having a misspent youth like the majority of the people I had met after leaving high school, so this was a phase that I went through to make up for lost time.

I met Kelly the day she moved in. The boys were all so pleased with her, and thought she would fit in. Her love of music was similar to ours, and she ticked all the important boxes. She had a job, she seemed nice, and wasn't bad looking. She had short black hair, almost a punk pixie do, with a long fringe that swept across her face, and wore a black jacket over a plain tee with jeans and boots that I would have loved to be wearing myself. Kelly was an artist, one of those talented people who can draw what they see, as if it was a photo. She had a studio where she painted, and she was enrolled at the Queensland College of Art, the same place I had been three years earlier.

We became friends instantly. In the beginning, our afternoons were spent on our veranda smoking cigarettes and drinking beer while dissecting our days at work. We worked similar shifts, and she came along to my art classes each week, which brought me a whole new appreciation for drawing.

Kelly was the first of us to leave for work each day, jumping into her car in the dark to make her way to the north side of the city. She was so generous and kind-hearted. The boys and I knew we could text her to bring home anything we needed, from milk, beer, smokes, and bread to a random veg for dinner. We knew it was no trouble because she didn't mind. She had a car and zipped around the city, unlike the rest of us, who walked, rode our bikes or caught the bus.

As the months went on, I noticed Kelly seemed to be going through a rough patch. She was tired, her smiley face was not as vibrant as it once had been and her eagerness to help had toned down. It was as if she was dragging her feet, and I felt a change in her. Something wasn't right. I wrapped my arms around her and gave her a big hug, knowing that she needed one. It was just us girls in the house, so we took the opportunity to recreate those early days on the veranda, beer in hand as we rolled our smokes.

She explained to me how the people at work kept her back most days by asking her to do longer hours, extending her shifts by up to five hours. She was torn because, yes, she wanted the money, but she was also quickly becoming exhausted.

Her mum had also reached out to Kelly for help. She had so much work piling up and she wasn't getting through it. Kelly felt bad so, after her shifts, she drove over to lend a hand to her mum for several hours, helping out with her work or her brother.

While all this was coming out, I could sense that she had taken on too much. Her generosity had been taken advantage of. She continued to share how some days she just wanted to come home and relax, and the last thing she wanted to do was drive someone to the shop or pick up supplies on her way home.

'Hey Kel, so why don't you say no?' I asked her.

She started to explain how it was her way of contributing to the house because she was so grateful to live here with all of us. Tears began to well in her eyes. Our house felt like a community, family and home, something I resonated with deeply. It was the first place where I felt I really belonged. I loved that she was happy to be here but I reassured her that she didn't need to be our doormat and do all the things she had been doing for us. It wouldn't make us like her any less. We all loved her and respected her for who she was. Now that I understood her situation, I went into battle to control who was asking what of her.

I remember giving her a pep talk to calm her worry. 'Remember what is important. Just say no. It will feel hard, but if you keep saying yes, everything will stay the same here, at work, and with your family. Stand your ground – you don't need to explain yourself. A NO is enough! You've got this.'

A simple no was all she needed; no excuses or justifications. Over the course of the following week, I saw her attitude change. Kelly turned down extra hours so she could help her mum, because that felt more important. And I cheered her on for it!

Thursday clocked around, and I had come down with the flu. I was feeling rough around the edges and I had an art class to run. I wanted to see if Kelly could cover me for the night. As a fellow artist, she had done it once before.

I waited for her to walk through the door to ask her in person. I met her in the kitchen as she put her bag down. My face was red, snot running out of my nose, with a fever. I had enough proof to appeal to her that I was in no way pretending, and really needed a favour. So I asked, 'Hey Kel, would you mind covering me tonight for art class?'

And you know what she said?

She said no!

I was totally bummed out. Why had I taught her the power of saying no!? I needed a favour! Seriously, how could this be happening? I was so sick.

EMPOWERMENT THROUGH BOUNDARIES & PROTECTION

It took me about two seconds to realise what she had done. Standing there, I smiled hard at her as I waited for her to witness her own courage. She was nervous and awkward, and I probably confused her more with my smile.

I wrapped my arms around her and said, 'Do you know what you just did? You said no, Kel! Congratulations!'

'I feel really bad,' she said. 'I hate letting you down.'

'Don't worry. I'll be fine. I am so proud of you for sticking to your guns.'

What happened over the following months was a silent revolution. Kelly stood her ground, and her smile returned. That evening in the kitchen was a bittersweet moment for me, but I loved that I was the person that got to share the power of no with her – and be the recipient of it as well.

The reason I understood her predicament so well is the old saying, 'It takes one to know one'. I did things for others to make them happy too and to show my gratitude. I felt like giving was my way of paying back my debt for other people's kindness.

I didn't know it back then, but I can see it for what it is now: a dead giveaway that we both were approval seeking.

What if, instead of holding worry close to our hearts, we got to choose how we spread our kindness? What if we let go of needing to prove that we can, and instead honour what is important to us?

It's a powerful moment to say no for the first time.

The uncertainty of what might happen next can buckle our knees, and make us just say yes, when we really mean no. The energy shift is subtle each time we deny ourselves an opportunity to speak our truth. We feel the emotional ramifications, and our energetic body stores and holds on tight to the weight, waiting for an outlet, while it secretly simmers out the last of our unique zest for life.

No is power.

No without explanation is power.

No because you prioritise yourself is power.

No because you have chosen to honour who you are is magic.

Say YES only when you really mean it.

HOW TO SAY NO WITHOUT THE GUILT

Resist the urge to justify or overexplain yourself	TRY: • Thanks, but I'll have to pass. • I can't today. • No, thank you. *(Remember to keep it simple and to the point.)*
Refer them	TRY: • Unfortunately, I can't; however, you could try {insert person for them to contact}. • I know someone who would be perfect for this. *(Remember this is helping the person find the best person for the job.)*
Know your limitations	TRY: • Unfortunately, I don't have time for that today. • I'd like to help, but I can't manage that at the moment. *(It's important to be aware of our personal resources: time, money & energy)*

EMPOWERMENT THROUGH BOUNDARIES & PROTECTION

Be persistent	TRY: Reinforcing your response over and over again until they get it. This takes courage, holding your ground. Eventually, they'll get the message. • Them: 'Can you help me get to work?' • You: 'Unfortunately, I can't.' • Them: 'You can pick me up at whatever time suits you?' • You: 'I can't today.' • Them: 'What if I cover your petrol money?' • You: 'Unfortunately, I still can't.'
Offer a counter solution	TRY: • I can't help you with that, but I can do *this* for you instead. *(Remember this is negotiating to find a middle ground that works for everyone.)*
Give yourself more time to respond	TRY: • Can I let you know in {insert time frame of choice}? • I'll put some thought into it and get back to you. *(Setting a time frame holds you accountable to come back with an answer – it's not to palm off the request.)*
Write yourself a permission slip	TRY: • I'm honoured you've asked, but I can't. • Thank you so much for thinking of me, but not today. *(Remember you have the right to make the best choice for you.)*

DEALING WITH BOUNDARY PUSHERS

Boundary pushers, or energy vampires, are people who are used to getting their way. They aren't used to people standing their ground and saying no. We need to remain strong in our fight to protect ourselves and keep our boundaries in place.

Navigating resistance is important for our mental and emotional well-being. This is the reason we are setting a boundary in the first place, right?

So what can we do about it?

- Repeat your response/statement to reinforce what you have just said. Perhaps you need to say, 'I can't today, maybe tomorrow' three times until the person gets it. This wears down the boundary pusher, as they love using your words against you – stick to the point and repeat. Don't budge.
- Is there a way you could negotiate? True compromise isn't abandoning your needs to please someone else, but finding a middle ground that works for both people. An example might mean instead of me instantly going to work for 6am, I say that I will be in at 8am, so that I have time for a shower, etc.
- Some people just won't respect your boundaries. We can't change someone else's behaviour, but we can choose whether to accept it, or to disengage.
- Circle back and try again – perhaps the timing was off, or the environment wasn't supportive of a conversation.

EMPOWERMENT THROUGH BOUNDARIES & PROTECTION

Dealing with people who want to test our boundaries is difficult, but it is also a gift. It's helping us to stand up for what we believe in, and it's tough at times. But when we start to make headway, and practise this new art, our confidence grows, and the guilt that used to consume us starts to wane.

Dealing with negative responses opens up an opportunity for us to try again. How can I communicate that boundary better so the other person understands what I'm asking of them?

Perhaps you need to revise your strategy; is there a better way to approach the situation? Can you adjust what you are asking for to find common ground? Perhaps you need to dig your heels in, and repeat your answer over and over, until they hear your 'no'.

ONE-LINERS!

For the people in your life that really push your buttons, it's time to arm yourself with some classic one-liners.

They need to be clear, concise, and honest. There needs to be no finger pointing. Just stating the facts.

Examples:

- *I'm sorry, I'm busy that day*
- *I've set boundaries around that; I hope you understand*
- *I'm comfortable with where I stand on this*

Boundaries protect your energy and life force. Don't see them as a negative, see them as an opportunity to educate the people around you about how you want to be treated. There should be no guilt in putting your needs first. If that pops up again, go back and address those fears. Is it due to your assumption, or fear, of how someone else is going to react? That really needs to be explored. Obviously, keep yourself safe at all times when setting boundaries; sometimes support is required to help you get a message across. In the next chapter we are going all in on communication, to help you find the words you need.

Chapter Ten
JUST ASK FOR IT

I LOVE GOING TO WEDDINGS, and this one was at a snazzy resort by the seaside. It was the first wedding we had been to since our own. However, this time we had a small Isla in tow, and I was two months pregnant with Harlan. I felt far from glamorous in the midst of motherhood.

One thing I've always done is get myself a new dress for every wedding I go to. It's such a special occasion, and I like to look my Sunday best! It's an opportunity to frock up and have a little fun. The problem was that I was also in dire need of a bit of a wardrobe update to tackle this little vay-cay. Every woman's worst nightmare: I had nothing to wear!

The harsh fluorescent lights of the shopping mall were ghastly as I searched for the right store. I had come prepared with a list of all things I was going to need for our trip, and I was child-free, and shopping solo! It was a weird experience, not having to dote over my eighteen-month-old. I was nervous, and anxious because shopping has never been my strong suit. Usually, I find the first store that looks like it has what I need, then I zip in and out and think nothing of it.

One pair of black trousers, check.

One white shirt, check.

Ah, perfect, now it's home time, and I can escape the madness.

Here, I was searching for that one shop in that exact frame of mind. I had my list, and I just had to go in and get the hell out.

Scared off easily by sales assistants, I would scope each shop before I went in to check the vibe. Most of the sales staff looked fake to me and just needed to earn a commission on what I bought, so of course they would say everything looked great on me! I hated looking at row after row, store after store, just to find a pair of jeans.

Finally, I found what I was looking for: jeans, T-shirts and even cool dresses in the shop window. I had struck gold. Walking in, I prepared myself for the moment the sales assistant pounced on me with a 'Hello, can I help you with anything?' Their enthusiasm frightened me. I simply smiled and blurted out, 'Just looking, thanks,' as quickly as I could. (Honestly, why do they have to do that? Give a girl some space!)

The loud upbeat music did nothing for the wave of anxiety that started to engulf me. My heart beat faster, encouraging me to hurry up and get this over with, so I could get out of the store, stop sweating, and flee back to the safety of my car.

Shopping feels like a battle of how to present yourself

to the world. Every store has its own size guide, constantly reminding us that we are inferior, and making us question who we are once we step inside the changing room. No wonder we struggle with body image!

Here I was, standing in the store's fitting room with a handful of possibilities to try on. It felt like years since I had done this. The full-length mirrors were unavoidable, emphasising my body's shape. I was trying not to break into a sweat on the clothes, only to be disappointed that the jeans I was trying to pull up were not getting past my thighs.

I felt doomed. It was a totally pointless exercise. I was fucking pregnant again, and even if I wasn't showing yet, having one child had already changed my body. Now I had giant fucking boobs, and an ass to match, plus the extra wobbly bits in between. The size 14 jeans that I was wearing had stretched out enough over the past two years to be the size that was my new normal, but the ones I was trying on didn't fit. Deflated, I thought, *What is the use? My body is going to change shape again, anyway. I've got a nice dress back home that will do for the wedding.*

Why would I spend money on clothes now when I probably wouldn't fit into them again, ever? I decided I shouldn't buy anything now, just wait until after I had my son and lost a few kilos before trying again.

Beyoncé started playing over the speakers, which took me out of my head for a moment. I loved this song. Then out of nowhere came a knock on the changing room door. If it wasn't bad enough that I had a pair of jeans halfway up my legs, jumping around trying to pull them up, the soccer field lights were just highlighting my discomfort from every angle. I could see my ass hanging out directly in front of me, thanks to all the mirrors! Damn that pesky sales assistant! *Here we go, people*, I thought, preparing myself for the onslaught of fake praise. *Yep, I look so good, blah blah blah.*

'Do you need help with anything?' she asked.

'Ah, I'm fine.' I quickly wriggled out of those jeans and went back to the pile to change the size.

Again with the knocking, she asked, 'Are you sure I can't help you in there?'

For fuck's sake, why was she back? 'No, I'm fine. Thanks!' I responded in my sweetest voice. I didn't want to be rude. It was as if I had someone breathing down my neck who wouldn't leave me alone. Becoming more flustered by the whole experience, I was no longer convinced that this was going to be the straight-in-straight-out, easy task that I had imagined. My need to demonstrate that I was a seasoned shopper, to prove to the sales assistant that this wasn't my first rodeo, was one hundred per cent a lie. I was more concerned that I was taking up all her time and attention.

I remember taking a good hard look at myself. I don't think I had seen my whole body before – this was before I had done the whole 'walk naked' experiment. Our small bathroom mirror over our sink was pretty much there to make sure we didn't have anything stuck in our teeth. In that moment, I saw it all, and my instant response was to mentally tear my whole body apart, from my tired panda eyes to my swollen feet. I could only see the bad. I tried to pull myself together and reminded myself that I was there to get a few things that would make me look and feel good for my weekend away.

Instead, I was full of self-loathing.

It was pointless.

I was ready to break down and have a good cry. I secretly think that Beyoncé song saved me a little. Something had to change.

Fuck it.

I surrendered, even though I had brushed the sales assistant off for a second time. My jeans were unbuttoned, my T-shirt was on the ground, and it was just me and my daggy bra and undies, in a mess of clothes, trying to win at shopping. I felt guilty for being there. I felt bad because I was out of my depth. I didn't want to admit I needed help. I desperately wanted to prove to myself that I could do this.

I peeked through the door to see if the lady was about. Grabbing her attention with my head popping out of the cubicle, she rushed over.

'I need help,' I finally admitted, to myself as much as to her. I went on to over-share my situation: the wedding, needing a dress, kids, being pregnant, and that I wanted to feel good. Within seconds she came back with a pair of jeans, a dress I would never have picked out, and a few other things.

I had dropped my guard.

All of a sudden, I was vulnerable and under her spell.

I surrendered all control to this beautifully presented woman, with her full face of make-up, cute dangly earrings, and carefully curated outfit. Her nails were done, and she wore heels! Like, wow! She looked good – far from how I was feeling.

Over the course of the next thirty minutes, I built a pile of clothes that I liked wearing. It just took me a moment to get over myself, and the bullshit I was saying in my head, to realise that the world was not out to fuck me over.

I had all the signs of an approval seeker:

- I didn't want to bother the sales assistant, even though she was there to help.
- I didn't want to feel uncomfortable or judged because I didn't like what I saw in the mirror.
- I wanted to prove that I could clothes-shop because I didn't want to seem weak.
- I assumed all sales assistants were judging me; I wanted their approval.

After I pushed my pride, stubbornness and desperate need to prove that I could do this alone to the side, I finally saw the situation for what it was. I had lucked out with a super helpful sales assistant, who could help me rock my curves, which made me feel like a total superstar. I had everything I needed for my weekend away, and I didn't feel guilty about my purchases, because I felt confident in the clothes that she had helped me to pick out.

I had asked for help!

It's a huge deal for approval addicts to do this, because we want to be seen as strong, competent, and able. Speaking up for ourselves is like a foreign language we have not learnt. In this chapter I'm going to give you all the tools to express yourself and create healthy relationships with people through effective communication.

THE CONSEQUENCES OF STAYING SILENT

Just imagine how that dressing room dilemma would have gone if I had not opened up and asked for what I needed. Well, I can tell you, because I've done it a thousand times before. I walk into that changing room, try on about ten things, and walk out empty-handed, feeling defeated, only to repeat it in the next shop, and the next. Leaving me feel like a failure, because it's something that I struggle with. I just want clothes to wear, so I resort to finding a shop with everything, settling for the closest thing to do the job. I do like comfort, but there is something to be said about a dress that fits well, especially if you are curvy like me, because no one wants to wear a sack to a wedding.

When we are silent, we are pushing down all of our emotions and feelings, which tells our body that they are not valid. Thus we create a pattern of autopilot behaviour that reconfirms whatever our inner bitch is saying – my personal favourite is *I'm not enough*. The cloud gets heavier and heavier. Until frustration is met with – *I can't do this anymore.*

Holding it together for someone else is a form of people pleasing. As approval seekers, we want to make sure we are displaying the correct emotion or reaction to someone else. This is why we have a whole chapter on communication.

Working with couples, and also improving my own marriage, the key to healthy relationships is learning to communicate and share our needs. A lack of communication sees both parties relying on assumption (the devil). Most relationships fall apart when something small is not resolved and is hung on to for years – like my husband doesn't help, or my wife is overly emotional. A small fracture, when held in silence, becomes bigger and more painful.

For those fellow 'overly emotional' types – that's me too – don't worry. I want you to imagine an empty cup – each time you have a rise of emotion, be it frustration, upset, anger or sadness, and you brush it off as nothing, I want you to add a stone to that cup. You get to take a few out if you have been practising how to move or express your emotions. But for now, let's assume you haven't. Each time, that cup gets fuller. It might take days, months, or even years. But there will be a point where something just tips us over the edge, and all hell breaks loose. Remember my kitchen incident with my husband?

It happens because we haven't spoken up. We've stayed silent.

While we are holding all that extra weight, we become drained from lugging it around, forcing niceties with those around us.

When we speak up, we are sharing the issue, which opens up more possibilities and ways to see the situation.

As approval seekers, we are hard-wired to be independent and do things for ourselves, because we don't want to come across as weak. Once upon a time, as a child, asking for help was something I felt uncomfortable doing, as it often resulted in feeling guilty and inadequate. This fear of being judged would result in struggling in silence to persevere.

We all want to succeed, but we don't know everything, so we need to learn, right? In order to learn, we need to be shown, and for that to happen, we need to ask.

We might feel uncomfortable, or weak at the thought of admitting our lack of knowledge or ability. But I want you to see it as a way of gaining information. And having more information is good, as it helps us to make more informed choices and decisions.

Asking for help builds trust.

POWER OF COMMUNICATION

The reason why so many of us find it so hard to express ourselves or ask for what we want is that we don't have the communication skills to do so.

Communication is not something that is taught in school. Yes, we can all read and write, but having adult conversations wasn't a subject any of us took. Instead, we were taught to respect authority, and to play by the rules.

Standing up for yourself was seen as the act of a rebellious child. Not a good one! And we were all taught that we needed to be good.

Many approval seekers alter the truth to accommodate others while shutting down their own feelings to survive. Concern about others' reactions become an obsession. Which leads them to feel unsafe when it comes to communicating their needs.

So, lots of us prefer to stay silent.

Sayings like, 'If you have nothing nice to say don't say anything at all' still live in my bones. What I've worked out is that delivery matters, and being honest strengthens relationships.

When we communicate with confidence, we are unstoppable, because we understand that everyone has a point of view, and that it's okay to be wrong, it's okay to be different and it's okay to be yourself. A total super power if you ask me. If I could go back to my younger self, the thing I wish I had learned is how to communicate more effectively. Being blunt and to the point has its advantages, but it stopped me from going under the surface to gain a deeper perspective.

Journaling has been the best tool to help me find my voice. To say things that feel a little naughty, because sometimes we really do want to call someone a fucking dickhead. But don't. Years of bottled-up thoughts and feelings are waiting to erupt. So putting them down on paper helps us to see them; it helps us to see our emotions and our thoughts in fact form. It invites us to explore how to problem-solve the situation and to ask, 'What is my truth in the matter?'

Once we find our voice on paper, we can articulate it better. This in turn means that we can ask for what we want, set boundaries, address discomfort or solve problems with ease, because there is no more hiding.

Journal Prompts

- *Which conversations do I tend to shy away from or struggle with?*
- *Why do I stop myself asking for help or for what I want?*
- *How comfortable am I with expressing myself?*

THE ART OF EFFECTIVE COMMUNICATION

I've been a great listener for years, but when it came to sharing my feelings, I would shut down, mostly out of fear of the dreaded rush of tears that would accompany me trying to get my words out. My emotions felt so big that words couldn't live alongside. I found it was easier to cry than to communicate. And that totally sucks for the other person, because they are left wondering what the heck has just happened and what they can do to help.

Ah… communication skills were required.

A conversation between two people is an energetic dance; it should flow with ease and compassion. There are a few key elements required for healthy conversations, including empathy, vulnerability, and curiosity.

Effective communication is being able to speak honestly from the heart.

There are many parts to master, such as what words to say, our tone, and how to listen instead of assuming.

FIVE ESSENTIALS FOR GOOD COMMUNICATION

Presence

To have meaningful conversations we need to be in our bodies, in the present moment. This allows us to listen to our body and observe our thoughts in real time. Having this openness allows us not to get caught up in the mind, but to show up for the other person, without distractions.

Being present in the conversation means you are investing in it, giving it the time it requires. When we do this, the other person can feel it, and can connect at an energetic level. There is more focus on the words being said, observing ourselves and the other person. This allows for a deeper experience.

By slowing down, we are grounding ourselves, calming our nervous system, which helps us to respond rather than react. It allows us to tackle questions and statements as they come.

MANTRA: Awake Body, Tender Heart, Open Mind.

Listening

The key to being a great listener is to encourage the speaker. This does not mean showering the other person in flattery. It's about keeping the conversation going and pulling out the details to really understand what the other person is saying. Listening requires questions.

To truly listen to someone, we need to ensure that they know we are hearing what they are saying. We need to avoid jumping ahead and assuming what they are going to say next. Instead, we need to respond to what they are actually saying.

Listening requires patience.

When someone opens up and starts sharing, we lean in with curiosity, but for most of us what we are searching for is a problem, so we can help 'fix' it for our friend, so they feel better because that's what good friends do; we hate seeing our loved ones in pain. This is where we might rush the conversation and not gain all the facts.

Inviting someone to share more is relatively simple. You can use phrases like: *tell me more, what happened next, how did it make you feel* and then pause, allowing them space to continue. The feeling of getting everything off your chest is one I love; it's like the heaviness has been lifted.

While listening and gathering information, it's important to clarify what's been said. This is crucial for heated or hard discussion, so they don't get misinterpreted. To do this, all you need to do is to reflect back what the other person has said – for example, while I was in the changing room with the sales assistant, I spoke about the wedding and the importance of having a dress, as I listed off several other things. She then said, where and when is the wedding? I continued to rattle off more information about the wedding – it was at the seaside in two weeks. I pointed out that I liked the look of the dress in the window, and she then asked me if I would like to try it on. It felt like she had read my mind, but she was letting me lead the conversation, by asking questions.

In therapist language, we call this active listening and clarifying. We want the whole lot, all the information.

Highlighting an important piece of information helps the person who is talking to expand on it, but also dig deeper too. It benefits both parties. For example, while asking all the things in the changing room, the sales assistant said, *You mentioned jeans?* I know it sounds simple but it led me to explain more about the jeans. She also asked a few questions to find out more about what exactly I was looking for.

Reflecting back what another person says feels super ridiculous when you first start doing it. I'm not going to lie. If your partner says, 'Want to go for lunch?' then you say, 'Did you say go out for lunch'? It's like you have gone deaf, but that is not the case at all. I want you to start confirming what the other person has said (this is a part of active listening). It's not just sitting and nodding, it's actively confirming their words. It's powerful, and it's a real game changer.

Speaking

When we speak and share our point of view, it's important to come across as calm (present) with a full understanding (listening) of the situation.

Our words have a profound impact on others. Just think about the things that were said to you as a kid; which ones do you believe now? In which situations did you feel seen and heard? When did someone share a story of wisdom to help you that was perfect in that situation?

Words pack weight. It's important for us to set the tone before we speak.

During a conversation, we should be asking loads of questions. This is a practice in itself. From a person who likes to save the day, and offers advice, solutions or problem solving, it's important to find out if the person you are listening to wants that.

It's your sense of duty to respond carefully. You could ask, *Would you like to hear what I think? Do you know what I would do? Would you like to hear my opinion? What can I do to support you?*

If you are opening up for the first time to share your own experience or feelings, it's important to remember to take ownership of them. To know what you want from the conversation. Perhaps you need to address a situation that is a little delicate. What needs to be said. Big conversations require us to be true to ourselves, not blaming or shaming one another. *You did this, You did that* should be turned into *I was uncomfortable when this happened and I would like it more if we could do this.*

This is why I find writing so powerful; it has helped me to have those big conversations and to work out what I want from them.

Our words matter; make sure you are using them wisely and compassionately.

Openners

We can't control others; we don't know what other people are thinking, or their beliefs or opinions unless we ask them. With all communication, there is the unknown. This is not to be feared, but met with curiosity.

Bravery is speaking our truth and allowing it to land for others. How they respond is on them. It's a result of their own internal make-up. It doesn't mean that there is anything wrong with us or them.

Being open to others allows the conversation to flow with ease. It's removing any judgement and accepting the current words in the present moment. We get to honour our courage, no matter the response. We may not get the result we want but…

You never know what speaking your truth can unfold for you unless you do it.

Responding

Understanding ourselves comes with time, practising our communication takes dedication, and handling what others throw at us takes courage.

Life is a game. And I want you to sign up with love. What if we…

- respond to fear by offering support
- respond to loneliness by connecting
- respond to pain with compassion
- respond to grief with comfort
- respond to anxiety with action
- respond to happiness with celebration

What would happen? Meet each interaction with compassion, openness, and a willingness to listen before responding, and see how the world changes in front of you.

We have a choice about how we respond – make it matter.

Five Tips to Improve Your Conversations

- Practise pausing and waiting for a response, instead of trying to fill the gap.
- Be confident when you ask/state what you need. Your energy is powerful, so get in the right frame of mind to take on big conversations.
- Walk into a conversation without any expectation – don't let assumptions and judgments cloud your mind – be open.
- Start small and move on to bigger conversations as you become more confident in asking for what you want (move through the discomfort).
- The art of communication is a practice; keep at it because it's a valuable tool to get more of what we want.

SCRIPTS FOR BIG CONVERSATIONS

Big Conversations can feel daunting, but with clear communication, we can navigate these moments with confidence, clarity, and kindness. This section provides practical scripts to guide readers through some of life's most difficult discussions, empowering them to ask for what they need, set boundaries, and handle sensitive topics without over-explaining or apologising.

Asking for What You Need Without Over-Explaining or Apologising

It's happened to all of us. 'I'm so sorry to ask you this but I just need...' Perhaps we go on to justify why we are sorry after asking for what it is we need.

Asking for something should not come with an apology. It's almost as if we aren't giving the other person a choice, and hope that they buy into the story instead of being honest. It's almost as if we are saying, 'Hey, I have no choice,' instead of asking because we want something.

This can dilute the message and weaken the ask. The key is to be clear, direct, and concise.

WHAT NOT TO DO:

'I'm really sorry to ask, but I'm struggling to find something to wear. I know you're busy, but do you think you could maybe help me? I totally understand if you can't.'

CONFIDENT SCRIPT:

'Hi there, I'm looking for [specific thing], can you point me in the right direction?'

Key Phrases for Asking Without Apologising:

- 'I need your support with…'
- 'Could you help me…?'
- 'Could you take on [task]?'
- 'Let's discuss how we can…'

Setting Boundaries and Standing Up for Yourself in Relationships

Setting boundaries can feel uncomfortable, especially if you're worried about how the other person will react. But boundaries are essential for maintaining healthy relationships. A clear boundary expressed with kindness and firmness will go a long way.

What not to do:

'I'm sorry, but I just can't handle helping you all the time. It's starting to really stress me out. I hope you understand that I need some time for myself.'

Confident script:

'Unfortunately, I'm unavailable, but I could help you on [day/time] if that suits'

'I want to continue to support you, but I need to take care of myself too. I can help you at the weekend when I have more time and energy. I hope you understand.'

Key Phrases for Setting Boundaries:

- 'I'm unable to [task] right now, but I can…'
- 'I need to focus on myself, and I can't commit to

[task] at this time.'
- 'I'm happy to help within these limits…'
- 'I value our relationship, and to maintain it, I need…'

Setting boundaries firmly but respectfully allows the other person to understand your limits without guilt-tripping or resentment.

Conversation Starters for Sensitive Topics

Difficult topics, such as asking for a raise, discussing personal feelings, or addressing conflict, require both sensitivity and clarity. Here are scripts to initiate these conversations with care.

What not to do:

'I hate to bring this up, but I've been working really hard, and I was wondering if it would be possible to discuss a raise. If not, I understand, but I thought I should ask.'

Confident script:

'I've been contributing to the team's success in [specific ways], and I believe it's time to discuss and review my salary?'

What not to do:

'I don't want to make you feel bad, but I've been feeling like we don't spend enough time together lately. I know you're busy, so if you can't, I totally understand, but it's been bothering me.'

Confident script:

'I've been missing spending quality time together, and it's something that's really important to me. Can we talk about finding time to connect more, even if it's just small moments throughout the week?'

What not to do:

'I don't want to start a fight, but it really upsets me when you do [specific action]. I don't know how to bring it up, but it's been bothering me a lot.'

Confident script:

'I want to talk about something that's been on my mind. When [specific action] happens, I feel hurt, and I'd like to find a way for us to address this so we can avoid it in the future.'

What not to do:

'I don't think the way you're handling the kids is right. You're either too strict or too lenient, and it's frustrating for me.'

Confident script:

'I've noticed we have different approaches to handling [specific situation with the kids]. I think it's important we find a balance that works for both of us. Can we discuss how to align our parenting styles better?'

What not to do:

'I know this happened a long time ago, but I'm still really hurt about it. I don't think you understand how much it affected me.'

Confident script:

'There's something from the past that I haven't fully processed, and I think talking about it now could help me move forward. Can we revisit this and find a way to heal together?'

What not to do:

'Your family is really getting on my nerves, and I'm tired of dealing with them all the time. I don't think they respect our boundaries.'

Confident script:

'I really value our time with your family, but I've noticed some situations that make me feel uncomfortable. Can we talk about how to set healthier boundaries so both of us feel more at ease?'

Handling Big Conversations with Confidence

Stay calm and grounded: If emotions start to escalate, take a moment to breathe and ground yourself before continuing.

Focus on 'I' statements: Speak from your own experience rather than blaming or accusing. This helps maintain a constructive tone.

Practise ahead of time: If it's a particularly tricky conversation, rehearse your key points to ensure you stay on track.

Be clear and concise: Get to the point without over-explaining. This shows confidence and respect for the other person's time.

F*CK APPROVAL, YOU DON'T NEED IT!

Listen actively: After you've expressed yourself, allow the other person space to respond. Conversations are two-way streets.

Phrases for Navigating Tricky Discussions Confidently

SITUATION	WHAT NOT TO SAY	TRY THIS...
DECLINING AN INVITE	'I'm really sorry, but I don't think I can come to your event. I feel so bad about it.'	'Thanks for inviting me. I won't be able to make it, but I hope you have a great time.'
GIVING NEGATIVE FEEDBACK	'I don't want to upset you, but I feel like you're not pulling your weight.'	'I'd like to talk about how we can improve our teamwork. I've noticed [specific issue], and I think we can address it by [solution].'
HANDLING CRITICISM	'I know I've made mistakes, and I'll try harder next time.'	'Thank you for the feedback. I'll have a think about it.'
SETTING A WORK BOUNDARY	'I don't think I can take on this project. I'm sorry.'	'I'm currently at capacity and won't be able to take on this project right now.'
EXPRESSING FEELINGS	'I don't want to make a big deal out of this, but it's been bothering me...'	'I need to share how I've been feeling so we can address it together.'

Chapter Eleven
MAGIC IN THE MUNDANE

SELF-TRUST GIVES US POWER. AFTER our very stretchy move to Scotland, I decided to give my intuition a run for its money. I'm talking about that gut feeling we often get when we know something is meant for us. It's fuelled by a deep desire. Like me, you may have pushed it down, because you thought it was too big, crazy, or wild. Maybe you didn't bring it up with the people around you because the fear of being judged was all too much.

The final piece of how to overcome approval addiction is to master trusting yourself.

My first experience of this was when I realised how much I needed mountains in my life. Six months later we were in a flat with the exact view I had been craving. Willingly going into such a big change, I left it to the universe to help. When I use the word universe, I think of it as 'divine timing' – most of us would say it's a sign that something is 'meant to be'. This requires us to trust our gut, and have faith that things will work out how we want them to.

F*CK APPROVAL, YOU DON'T NEED IT!

I held the vision.

I believed it fully, and felt deeply connected to it. It wasn't driven by ego, but by a feeling, delivered by a vision, while journaling, leaving a smile on my face. I understood my emotional and energetic body. This was a scream that I refused to ignore.

I trusted my magic to bring it to fruition.

When that happens, it's a total 'pinch me' moment. It took a while to soak in, because I was in disbelief. I had outside validation feeding my approval addiction, but it made me uncomfortable. That's because it's weird to celebrate; approval addicts just don't do that. But this was big.

I made magic happen.

This chapter is about how to turn the mundane into magic, learning how to celebrate our wins along with the art of receiving. You'll find my favourite rituals to deepen your relationship to self. Plus, I will leave you with my favourite mantra to invite the universe to send you more signs of expansion and fulfilment.

*

Sitting at the park while all the kids run wild after school is where I get my dose of socialising. Catching up with the other mums when the weather is fine enough for us to sit on the one park bench. We talk about all the things. Here I learned the difference between tights and stockings, how to pronounce a neighbouring town, along with how to navigate the latest kid drama.

To my surprise, one mum mentioned a lack of counsellors and therapists locally. I asked all the questions about what was on offer in the area. I wanted to help; silently I acknowledged this, while my head came in with a loud 'I can do that'. I was a qualified cognitive behavioural therapist (CBT) who loves psychology and seeing people improve their lives.

This little moment was very clear.

Something in me stirred. I spent the night talking it through with Roy. My practical man loves to ask me how it will all work, which totally killed my vibe. So I parked it.

A few days later we were attending a party for staff and families at Roy's work. I got to meet hubbie's work colleagues, have a few drinks and even try my hand at axe throwing. I loved it, by the way, it felt invigorating. A few people mentioned that they wished that they had someone to talk to, and I casually mentioned that I was a CBT. One of the loveliest women I met encouraged me to let her know when I would have sessions available.

Talk about signs! It was as if the universe had spoken.

Still hesitant that this would work, I created a Facebook post offering walking sessions to see if I would get any takers. Low risk. I had a feeling it would work. It wasn't going away.

Having slowly scaled back my online sessions for clients in Australia due to time-zone logistics, I was desperate to offer sessions in person, as much as for myself as others. I like the energy exchange that happens; I can read people as a whole, feel their energy, and dive deeper into conversations.

F*CK APPROVAL, YOU DON'T NEED IT!

Booking a couple of sessions, I was surprised by the number of enquiries. I began looking for a space to use. Scotland is unreliable when it comes to the weather, and for me to spill my guts on how I feel, I need a safe space. One that is warm! Within days I found something that would work. It wasn't ideal, but I had clients waiting for sessions.

After I'd used the room a couple of times and run the numbers, I was disheartened. I was making below minimum wage for my time. The space wasn't quite right. I had a dilemma to solve.

A few nights later I got cosy in bed and had a thought. *I swear there is a room on the second floor on the way up to the wool shop in the High Street.* Having kept my search going in all the normal avenues, I decided to follow this nudge. So I sent a message to the wool shop sheepishly asking if there was a room to rent in the building.

Three days I waited.

I was at a loss. Nothing else seemed to fit or was going to work. But I got a reply confirming that there was a room up for rent and to contact the landlord. The next day we spoke and decided to meet that Friday to see the room and its facilities.

Walking down the High Street to meet the landlord and the wool shop owner, I went over what needed to be discussed. It had what I needed: a secluded entrance, a toilet and most importantly a room that was private with good light. Taking the stairs up through the blue door, I soon surprised myself with the fact that the building only had two storeys. The room that I was going to look at was next door to the wool shop, and when I looked through the door, I smiled.

What I saw was a room with two big windows with all the light coming in, a circle of couches and chairs, a few plants, and shelves of wool. I totally had a giggle to myself. You see, I didn't go and check to see if it actually had what I thought was there. I decided to trust this fully. If it was meant to be, it would have what I needed.

I fell in love. It was perfect.

I moved in a few weeks later and opened my CBT practice. It took a few weeks to come clean about my plans to the ladies in the wool shop. From that moment they got their first dose of Liz and my magic. I believe that what is meant for us will happen, when we trust ourselves. This is knowing ourselves inside out. Those thoughts that drop and land big are worth listening to. The feelings that sit alongside them help us to gauge their importance.

Some call it luck. But I call it magic.

There were loads of working parts that needed to come together to make this happen. I put myself out there in a big way. I wanted to see if the pieces would all fall into place, and the signs were clear that I was right where I needed to be.

Trusting your magic will open up opportunities aligned with your desires. This is where embodiment thrives in harmony with our mind. Call it self-belief. Aligned living.

Validation came that this was right, and I gave it to myself. I won. My approval addiction was no more. Life was now all kinds of magical.

I stopped seeking.
I started believing.
I trusted my magic.

BREAKING FREE FROM 'MEH'

If I had broken trust with myself, I would have fallen back into my approval addiction, seeking out validation from others. Starting a business is never easy, and to do it in a new place comes with its challenges. But it was clear that it was meant to happen, in my wee office. I made a choice to back myself.

Our choices signal a series of events to occur that either support us or have us wanting to turn back instantly. That is their power. Once we make a choice, that chain reaction begins unfolding, providing us with new information. In any given moment we can make a choice to stop, or to continue, to ask for more information, or a sign. Owning our choices puts us in the driver's seat; we are no longer waiting for someone else to tell us how to do something.

I've learned that there are many ways to do simple tasks. It's not just 'my way or the highway', that is a total limitation and has us living by someone else's rules. We want to transform our everyday 'meh' or mundane life into something a little more special. Because by now you have realised the importance of creating and maintaining your own happiness.

When I was a kid, my great-aunt came to stay with us for a night. We were putting pillow cases on her pillows to make up her bed, and she told me the way I was doing it was wrong. Taking this discussion out to the living area,

I mentioned it to my parents, and they suggested that we should have a race to see who could get the pillowcase on the fastest because that was the underlying issue; me flapping a pillow about seemed a little 'too much' for a young lady. Yes, I was wild.

Of course, I won; my great-aunt was so upset by this. She believed that it was far quicker to do it the 'correct way', which also ensured the pillow was in the correct position. But I walked away feeling pleased with myself. This lesson came back to me when Roy began doing the dishes in our house.

I don't mind washing dishes; I get to play in the water and play Tetris while I do it. The art of stacking had been developed in my earlier years when faced with a week's worth of dishes. Even as an unruly teenager, I would put on my favourite tunes and just dive in, and get the task done as quickly as possible. It was pretty clear that this not-so-glamorous task was mine for the rest of my life, having heard how my own mother had done dishes since she was young. A rite of passage, perhaps.

As much as there were times I really didn't want to do it, I found ways to make washing dishes more enjoyable. When Roy took over this job in our house, I wondered why it took him so long. A job I could smash out in fifteen minutes tops could take him anywhere up to forty-five minutes. No, I am not kidding.

Washing dishes is a mundane job.

I asked him why it was taking so long, and then he explained to me his method. I was like, what? Are you crazy? He individually washed each item, rinsing it off delicately before placing it on the drainer. There were a few accusations thrown around about who was in fact doing the dishes correctly. And then I remembered my great-aunt and the pillowcases. The moral of that story was that it doesn't matter how the pillow gets its case on, it just needs to be done. Just like the dishes; it doesn't matter how it gets done, just that it is done. That was important. In our house, dishes are always done in the evening. Everywhere we have lived there have been ants, and if you leave the smallest of scrap of food on a bench, those sneaky dudes march a highway to the spot, and work out how to dissect it to carry it back to their home.

I want to remind you that there are no rules for how you do mundane and 'meh' tasks. It's about completing the job. Do it in style, and in a way that works for you.

When Roy worked away from home, the task was all mine and I decided (I made a choice) to not hate doing it, but to make it a ritual. Even the dishes can get sexy. I would put on my washing-up gloves so the water could be super-hot, but my hands would be protected – the detergent did some sort of weird things to my skin. The tunes would be on, my apron securely in place for all the splashes. The dishwashing liquid was even scented of roses, so it felt a little luxurious. Stacking the pans and pots in an artful way to create sculptures, I would take the time to enjoy being on my own in the kitchen at the end of the day, especially after running around with two kids all day. It was a recalibration, a slowing down. I would often sigh, releasing the weight of the day. My moment of victory would be celebrated with a piece of dark chocolate, and cuddles on the couch with my kids.

Starting a task in a bad mood sees us throwing things about, often setting the scene for something to go wrong. Negative energy loves to be fed too, and it's important that we don't give it the satisfaction it is craving. This is why our thoughts are the first thing we need to address regarding our task ahead. Mindset matters. Accepting the task needs to be done, we can prepare ourselves. Just like clearing the runway for take-off, we are setting ourselves up for success. Remember back when I was living in the UK in my early twenties and I had to vacuum the floor of the house and take two hours doing it? I had to make my peace with the task and turn it into a more meditative exercise. It can be done. If you are still questioning whether your mind will get on board with the task, go back to Chapter Five, and start hacking your beliefs.

We all have to do a lot of the same things, day in and day out. My dad calls it SSDD – same shit, different day. From washing dishes, to taking out the garbage, to earning a living, to grocery shopping, and beyond. I want you to explore ways to make these tasks less 'meh' for you.

How can we make this fun, or at the very least bearable?

I've seen people outsource tasks that they don't have time for because of their busy work and life schedule. I've also seen people outsource tasks that they really don't like doing.

Perhaps you don't have the budget to make this happen. I want you to focus on getting your mindset on board, getting the job done, and making peace with the daily task. Sprinkle in the magic you require. I have a friend who watches rom-coms while making dinner. One of our neighbours would get dressed up to take the bins out, I swear! Always puts a smile on my face. I like doing some tasks with people as it makes it more enjoyable, while other times I'm happy for the solitude. And this is why knowing yourself inside out helps, because we can easily find solutions. It just takes a little creative thinking to turn the dread of mundane activities around. Honestly, we are currently looking at getting a dishwasher installed. Why not, hey?

Magic can happen in the mundane when you create rituals to support you, to set the tone of your life, to see the world through a lens of beauty. All it takes is for us to slow down, listen to our internal whispers, and go from there. The present moment matters.

Play with life; being bogged down limits our potential.

There will of course be times in our life where we fall apart, and it's not to prevent us from creating our dream life. Instead, it invites us to seek our truth, to understand when to nurture ourselves or how and when to take action.

You are in control of how you shape the world around you. Don't be a victim to the dishes or anything else. You have a choice.

Here are my favourite rituals for life.

RITUALS FOR LIFE

The Gratefuls

> 'Acknowledging the good that you already have in your life is the foundation for all abundance.'
> – *Eckhart Tolle*

A daily gratitude practice will help you to honour your experiences. This practice can be as elaborate or as simple as you like. Practising gratitude helps to regulate emotions, calms the nervous system, improves relationships, physical health and so much more.

This cute little practice has been in our house since our kids were super little. It was a way for us to get more out of them about their day. After seeing something similar at a birthday party, I rejigged it to work for us. Each night, over dinner we pass a golden buddha around the table to signal when it was someone's turn to share their 'grateful' from the day. We found using an object helped the kids to focus and understand whose turn it was to talk. It doesn't need to be a golden buddha, it can be a yellow Pokemon, a fluffy green dragon or a mini football. At first it took a little practice for our family to get used to this ritual. Now the kids ask us each day, no prompts required.

The use of a prop helps younger kids to practise being patient, and to get used to the spotlight. The prop works for adults too, especially at large get-togethers, as passing it on signals when the person has finished.

To help the kids first start this practice, I would ask them what their favourite part of the day was. Any act of goodness that they had experienced which brought a smile to their face.

How To:

Find an object in your house that represents gratitude. This could be a buddha, a rock, a feather, a flower – it needs to be easy to pick up and hold. Each evening at the dinner table, with your friends and family (whoever sits with you), take turns to hold the object, and share one thing you are grateful for from that day. Pass the object on to the person beside you once you have done.

Start by saying – 'I am grateful...' (fill in the blank).

It's harder than you think, trying to find the good in your day. Once you do, though, it will open your eyes to all the positive things that happen each day. This practice has infused our family with connection and understanding.

Want to take it deeper? We now let the kids ask questions of the person who has shared their 'grateful', fleshing out details and sometimes revealing a life lesson.

If you don't have company, spend five minutes reflecting over your day and write down a list of 'gratefuls' in a journal.

DAILY SELF-REFLECTION

This practice is a check-in, and it's one that I journal at the end of the day when I come through the door or before bed. I think of it as decompressing. An opportunity to get over the day's events, and let off any steam, or determine if I need to move any emotions that came up during the day. I start with the following four journal prompts and if I feel called, I will write out my whole day or scenarios that got under my skin.

- *How do I feel?*
- *What challenges did I face today? What emotions came along for the ride?*
- *What were my wins? My favourite parts?*
- *What did I learn about myself?*

CREATING A MORNING PRACTICE

This isn't your cue to get up at 4am. This is your invitation to start your day right, and to get you in the mood to slay your day. It's putting things in place to ensure that your vibe is where you want it to be. I love starting my mornings grounded and slow, and then about half an hour in, the tunes get turned on. Having high-vibe tracks playing often calls for impromptu dance parties, which in our house end up in fits of laughter.

Establishing a morning practice is about nurturing your essence and setting the vibration for the day ahead. Designing your own requires a few things. One, work out how much time you have to play with. Two, decide what is the feeling you are wanting to create. Three, what do you need to do to get that feeling?

Morning practices change as we do over time, and it's important to acknowledge the phase we are currently in and to determine what we need.

A grounding morning practice could look like: starting with a meditation in bed before getting up, a cup of tea by your favourite window while reading a book, followed by a nourishing breakfast.

If a high-vibe practice is called for, it could look like: setting the alarm early; singing in the shower to your favourite power ballads; picking out an outfit that makes you feel unstoppable, thinking also about hair, make-up, and accessories. Put on your fave tune while you make your green smoothie to go.

These are very different energies, so I want you to craft a morning practice to suit you and your needs. A normal work day requires something different from attending a wedding. So set the mood to start your day right. Play with a few things to see what fits.

CREATING AN EVENING PRACTICE

Sleep is one of our greatest assets; when we give our body the time to rest and recover, we can operate on all cylinders. This is why having an evening practice to support our sleep is essential. Night-time routines are not just for kids; we need them too.

The first thing I do when I'm adjusting or creating an evening routine is I work out how much sleep I need. We all need different things, and for me to function at my best I'm looking for a solid eight to nine hours; meanwhile my husband functions on about six. I honestly don't know how he does it. But if he sleeps longer he is more lethargic during the day and just doesn't seem like himself.

Work out how much sleep you need. Then, ask yourself what time you are getting up in the morning. If I aim to get up around 7am, that means I need to be in bed by roughly 10–11pm at the latest. This allows me enough time to get to sleep and wake up with ease.

What supports you getting a good night's sleep is the next question we need to address. Heavy blankets? No lights? I'm a no-device-or-phone-in-the-room person, I like quiet and a cosy bed. I make sure I have all those things to ensure that I get a good night's sleep. So, is your room ready for you to sleep?

Factoring in how long it takes you to get ready for bed, I want you to explore things to help you calm your nervous system, ready for a good night's sleep. If the tea you are drinking is making you wee 500 times during the night, perhaps swap it, try something new, or leave it.

Before getting into bed, I consider how I want this time when I am turning off my brain to look. Do I read a book, listen to a podcast, watch a bit of telly? Do I journal, do meditation, go for a walk or sit outside?

Write out your plan from bedtime backwards, what you need, and how long it should last, so you understand when to start your ritual. Make it lush – I love the minutes when I apply moisturiser, the smell followed by the coldness of the *gua sha* rock I use to slowly glide over pressure points on my face. It's a mini facial that tingles as I lie down. I love it.

THE LITTLE THINGS I DO FOR ME!

Self-care is about taking time to nurture our needs. Taking thirty minutes a day might seem a lot to some, while others have moved on to that not being enough. This is a starting point, to create a self-care ritual that means something to you. You can break it up by doing fifteen minutes in the morning and another fifteen in the afternoon, or do it in one chunk. But it needs to address what you need in the moment. It doesn't have to be nails and spa days. These things might work for some people, but they are not everyone's cup of tea.

Here is a list of scrumptious things you can do to create more magic in your life.

- *Applying moisturiser (honestly, who knew it was bliss)*
- *Going for a walk outside*

- Reading a book
- Crafting, painting, creating, sewing, knitting, drawing, colouring
- Playing an instrument, singing
- Dancing
- Taking a bath
- Massage
- Foot soak
- Listening to music
- Journaling
- Yoga, gentle stretching (look up Yin Yoga)
- Baking

CREATING A CELEBRATION PRACTICE

When you achieve something notable, getting an award, landing a contract, selling a house, whatever it is, I want you to celebrate.

Share the news with the people you love; these people want to see you winning in life. The ones that don't, you really need to ask about the quality of that relationship. Perhaps revisit the support system in chapter three.

I want you to gather one to five people that would happy-dance with you. Share the news and toast to your success. Ideas:

- Have them over for a celebratory drink
- Enjoy a meal
- Go out for dinner
- Attend an event
- Go out dancing
- Go and buy that dress you have been waiting to buy

Having your people around you to witness this moment helps you to cement it into your being. It won't just slip by as something else you have done. We deserve to remember it, so make it a moment worth remembering.

Yes Please, More Thank You.

It's so easy to keep running through life being busy, ticking off tasks, getting stuff done. But do you ever pause to acknowledge your achievements? Did I just make you uncomfortable again?

Travelling is my drug of choice; I love seeing expansive landscapes and it blows my mind at times how incredible this earth is. I stand in awe. Moved by my emotional response to what I am witnessing, I often shed a tear and think how lucky I am.

Living in the land of rainbows – that's Scotland – I started using a phrase that I would only use for the big stuff: Yes Please, More Thank You. I was introduced to this concept on a podcast by Jess Lively, in 2016, and used it as a way to celebrate when I got a contract, or sold out an event, or landed an opportunity that felt huge.

Celebrating my wins has always seen me calling Roy first to squeal with excitement, dance around on the spot, usually chanting 'OMG! OMG! OMG!' Then I would anchor that all with a squeal of delight – 'Yes Please, More Thank You.' The concept is brilliant. It's telling the universe you want more of that feeling, more of that experience.

Too often we brush off our big moments to look ahead to the next. I want you to stay in the magic of the moment for a little bit longer. Why? Because you deserve a little credit for achieving something, and when you spend the time sitting in celebration, it signals to your internal world that you want more too.

Celebrating can be uncomfortable, especially if you have never done it before. It really doesn't require anything too over the top. I've had a delicious home-cooked meal with a bottle of bubbly at the table to cheer a win. To talk about it and revel in my moment of glory with my family. I've also taken my husband out for a night of luxurious food to celebrate a milestone achievement. When we put in the effort, we deserve to be witnessed.

If having people saying nice things to us, or being the focus of an occasion seems a little much, I want to ask you, why is that, what is the story behind it? Do you really believe that someone should not celebrate their wins? Or is it just you who doesn't deserve to celebrate?

Ridiculous!

Celebrating yourself is a form of self-validation. Doing this builds up the muscle that you don't need others to tell you how great you are, but instead can see it for yourself.

Overcoming approval addiction and validating your dreams is rooted in deep self-trust. It's knowing that life lessons come your way to teach you, to test your rule book, and to give you a deeper understanding of self. It's an ongoing journey, to stretch and test yourself, to shift your focus on your needs and desires.

It's a call to stop waiting… to listen to your body's wisdom and know that everything is going to work out. Everything you need is within you. No one can tell you what you want for your life, so stop looking around you, stop looking to others to validate what you know is true.

It's time to trust yourself.

By now, you should have a greater understanding of yourself, how you have been playing a role that doesn't serve you. A role that has made it easy for others to get what they want from you, while you sacrifice your happiness to please them. That ends now.

You deserve to have the life you want.

You have the right to make that choice.

Stop worrying about what other people think, because it doesn't matter. They are not living your life, you are! So, stop asking if it is okay to do something. Because when you do, the first thing I want you to remember is…

FUCK APPROVAL, *you don't need it!*

ACKNOWLEDGEMENTS

FROM THE BOTTOM OF MY heart I am so grateful for the support and endless encouragement from my husband to bring this book to life. Roy, I love you, thank you for being my rock. My two kidlets, thank you for your patience while mummy was behind her computer for way too long. This book is for you, to remind you of your power and to stay true to it.

I want to say a huge thank you to my brutal AF, honest feedback giving friend Liz Lennon, without you this book would have made you cringe. I appreciate you to the ends of the earth for the hours of reading, proofing, editing and discussions to make this book what it is today. Another big thank you must go to Emily Krempholtz for helping me to master the art of storytelling and evoking emotions. You were there at the beginning, to help me get my words out, to complete a full manuscript. A true gift.

I also want to thank Carolina and Rosie, and the team at the Book Guild for believing in me and my book. A true partnership that is working for the greater good. Let's create some magic.

F*CK APPROVAL, YOU DON'T NEED IT!

Finally to my late grandmother, this book was written for you, a woman who only got to dream about adventure. I hope I did you proud, there are still so many places I am yet to go. Thank you for rooting me to my family and for the best chocolate cake recipe ever.

Made in the USA
Monee, IL
18 September 2025